Hemp for Migraine

How
CBD & Endocannabinoids
Prevent
Migraines

Jeremy Orozco

DISCLAIMER

I am not a doctor or nutritionist, nor am I your hemp guru or shaman. I am someone who has gathered vast amounts of migraine and endocannabinoid research to help you and your health care professional make informed decisions. I've included a disclaimer for people who are inclined to sue or make poor life decisions.

Legal Disclaimer

DEDICATION

I dedicate this book to those in search of research-backed methods of migraine elimination, because screw migraines.

CONTENTS

WHY I WROTE THIS BOOK

I never intended to become a migraine expert. Little did I know a call would change my perception of migraines and our medical system. An emergency is what firefighters refer to as a "call." Most people don't know that 90 percent of firefighter calls are not for fires, but calls for medical emergencies. Today, a good firefighter needs to be a great EMT or paramedic, but don't tell any of the old smoke breathers that.

Back to the call. I was taking the vital signs of an unconscious 40-year-old female when she abruptly woke up. Her speech slurred and one side of her face drooped, appearing paralyzed—signs of a stroke. The next few minutes of treatment could have determined the rest of her life. To our surprise, she irritably refused medical help and said, "I'm just having a migraine. It happens a lot. I go to the hospital, and they can't do anything about it."

Why couldn't doctors treat her migraines? Where could she turn for help?

I asked my wife's best friend, who is a trauma surgeon and migraine sufferer, "How bad is this problem?" She said that migraine drugs only work about 50 percent of the time for about half the sufferers who try them. The medications are far from a cure and often come with horrible side effects.

While modern medicine does incredible things for blunt trauma, bacterial infections, or conditions which can be visualized or monitored, hospitals are less successful at preventing invisible illness such as migraine, fibromyalgia, irritable bowel syndrome, Lyme disease, lupus, multiple sclerosis, hypothyroidism and other autoimmune conditions.

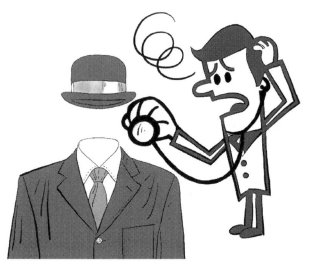

Something challenging to diagnose is often troublesome to treat and may come with social stigma from doctors, family, friends, and insurance companies, prompting sufferers to hide their invisible illness from the world.

Should you even see a doctor? Yes, you should talk to your doctor because you may have an underlying condition, such as a vitamin deficiency, that is responsible for all your migraine pain. Your doctor is your partner in the search for what's triggering your migraines. However, many migraineurs get nothing more than a migraine drug prescription and a pat on the back from their healthcare providers. Don't accept this from yours. Medications only mask the symptoms of migraines. The real way to eliminate migraines is with a strategy that reduces the underlying migraine triggers.

Unfortunately, the information that would help you create such a strategy is scarce and hard to find, so we (myself, my wife and her best friend—they are both MIT alumni, no big deal) decided to start a website for migraine help. We created a hub of the best migraine help. We collected thousands of migraine articles and resources. But it wasn't good enough. I became obsessed with finding the answer to migraines. My passion wasn't just for the good of others. It was personal.

My wife had occasional migraines, passed down from my mother-in-law who suffered chronic migraines. I had severe headaches and came to realize that the headache triggers responsible for my headaches were the same triggers causing my wife's and her mother's migraines.

During my search, I found that others had it much worse. According to the Migraine Research Foundation, migraine is the sixth most disabling illness in the world and the leading cause of all neurological disabilities.[1] About one billion people suffer from migraines. More than 90 percent of those sufferers cannot work or function during a migraine.[2] Migraines bring excruciating pain and high suicide rates. The stakes couldn't be any higher.

I discovered small clues in research that gave a glimpse into what was responsible for triggering migraines. I was fascinated by the measures that reduce migraines, because they were the same things that brought energy, health, and happiness. I had to know why there were studies that showed complete migraine remission, yet our medical system was failing migraine sufferers.

It was like I was on a boat that was sinking and people were slowly drowning below the deck. All I had to do was open a few doors, look for the holes, and patch them. The only problem was that opening those doors would expose the issues in a medical system that I worked within. I would need to jump off the ship to keep it afloat. I quit my job as a firefighter and followed those breadcrumbs for the last five years. It was worth it.

I systematically reviewed all the major migraine triggers and the most successful migraine studies. There was a commonality between all headache and migraine triggers, which I published in a 500-page book and on migrainekey.com. This commonality is the reason why the compounds in hemp are so useful in treating migraine. The same month my book was published, a breakthrough migraine study confirmed my findings.[3]

My wife no longer gets migraines. I was able to eliminate my headaches. My mother-in-law is entirely migraine free with only occasional headaches. Many of my readers have reduced or eliminated their migraines based on the same principles, which are published for free at migrainekey.com. Plus, these principles will also make you feel great.

The most disturbing thing I found was that our medical system is not designed to treat migraines. Migraine drugs are ineffective, in my opinion, and research is limited because migraine drugs don't make much money in comparison to the drugs for other diseases. In turn, the migraine education in our medical system is almost non-existent, which is a fact.

The average doctor only receives a total of four hours of education for all headache disorders, according to the World Health Organization.[4]

All Headache Disorders

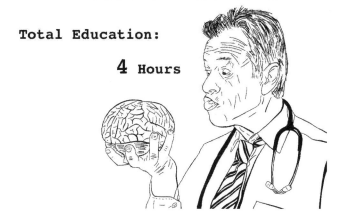

Total Education:

4 Hours

There are over 300 headache disorders and four hours of education to cover all of them. Neurologists only average one to five hours of total headache education. Many doctors have zero hours of migraine-specific education. It's hogwash. Are zero hours of migraine education acceptable for something that destroys 113 million workdays per year in the United States alone? This absurdity is not the fault of our doctors, but the system responsible for educating doctors and patients alike.

Only 40 percent of migraine sufferers are happy with their current treatment plan—but obviously would be more satisfied with a complete absence of migraine—according to a national survey of 3,900 migraine sufferers.[5] Studies show what triggers and reduces migraines, but most of this information doesn't cross the desks of our medical professionals. The most successful migraine studies are from natural substances and methods of relief. Hemp won't make it to our hospitals for the same reason it doesn't make it into mainstream medicine: hemp is absurdly cheap.

I'm excited about hemp because unlike migraine medications, it doesn't just mask the symptoms of migraines. Hemp has compounds that may attack an underlying trigger of migraines. The research in this book will show the power of hemp and how to amplify its effects. Positive testimonials are flooding in from migraine sufferers and we'll dissect the research that backs up their claims.

You deserve to know that a natural plant may do what our entire medical system cannot. This book isn't going to change how our medical system treats migraine, but sharing your personal experience could. Let's start a movement that could help up to one billion migraine sufferers.

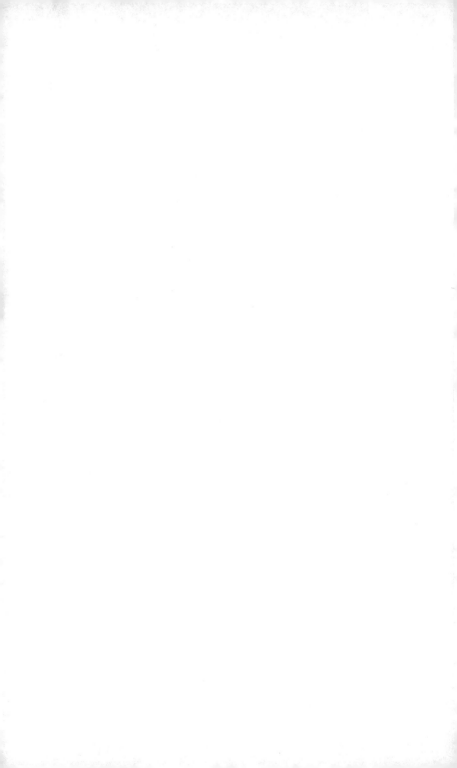

Part I: An Introduction to Hemp

HEMP WILL CHANGE MIGRAINE MEDICINE

There is a secret about hemp, which the government owns. Hemp contains neuroprotectants and antioxidants that are patented by the US government. They're called cannabinoids (*US Patent 6630507 B1*).[6] Cannabinoids are the reason why hemp is a breakthrough in migraine prevention and pain relief.

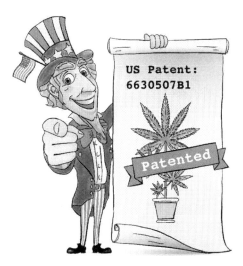

The most notable cannabinoid is called cannabidiol or "CBD" for short. CBD is best known for treating pain, nausea, anxiety, gut problems, sleep disorders, and epilepsy—making it your new best friend and a powerful compound to knock out migraines. The new research on CBD's neuroprotective qualities is equally impressive for migraine prevention.

If you're already taking notes, stop. Chill out. I've got you covered. The end of this book details how to get the Hemp for Migraine Guide Book, which summarizes all of the key points of the inspirational research found in Hemp for Migraine. I added the guide and a checklist to make it easy for anyone to succeed with cannabinoids and endocannabinoids, even those who are having trouble reading this book because their heads hurt. So, sit back and enjoy the ride.

Neuroprotection means protection of the neurons, which means protection of the brain and nervous system. Neurological disorders such as migraine, epilepsy, Parkinson's disease, and Alzheimer's disease are associated with neurological damage and therefore benefit from substances with neuroprotection.[7] That's the simple explanation anyhow.

The neuroprotection of CBD is so potent that studies on rodents have found that CBD not only prevents Alzheimer's damage, it can reverse cognitive deficits.[8] This is something that drugs have failed to do for Alzheimer's patients. The antioxidant properties that allow this neuroprotection to happen are what's vital for migraine prevention. Equally important, CBD doesn't come with the horrid side effects of most medications.

The best thing about CBD is that it does not get you high or stoned—I know that's a subjective opinion. Some cannabis strains contain CBD, but CBD itself does not elicit psychoactive effects. Most people don't realize that hemp may also contain CBD. In fact, CBD-rich hemp may benefit migraineurs who have not experienced relief from marijuana, because many cannabis strains are low in CBD or don't contain it at all.

Hemp is a type of cannabis that doesn't get you high. Most countries define hemp as any cannabis strain that has less than 0.3

percent THC. THC is psychoactive. THC is the cannabinoid that gets you high. THC is the reason that marijuana makes you feel like you are sinking into a chair, while your thoughts slowly drift away from your ambitions. At least that is what a friend tells me *(wink wink)*.

When a migraine strikes, you may want to use cannabis to numb your mind and body completely. However, most migraine sufferers need to stay sharp as a tack during the day-to-day hustle. Migraines already take a toll on mental clarity, which makes CBD an exciting treatment option. CBD calms the mind and body, without turning you into that person who asks midsentence, "What was I saying?" Later I'll also describe the ways to use THC for migraine prevention without it causing psychoactive effects, by either micro-dosing or using topical creams.

I began researching cannabinoids after my best friend told me that he used CBD to manage pain after surgery. We started as firefighters together. Recently, he sustained an injury on the job. He said he threw out his prescription opioids in preference of CBD drops from hemp, a bold claim. According to a study conducted by the University of California, his experience was not outlandish, but typical.

The University of California's research found that 97 percent of patients on opioid pain medication were able to decrease their opioid use with cannabinoids, and 87 percent of patients preferred only cannabinoids over opioids.[9] According to a sizeable survey reported in Forbes, nearly half of people who use CBD products stop taking traditional medicines such as opiates and other pain meds.[10]

The information is a breath of fresh air for migraine sufferers because hospitals prescribe opiates to migraine sufferers more often than migraine medications.[11] Migraine is not approved for opioid use, but in fairness to doctors, the other migraine drugs are not all that effective. Both opioids and acute migraine medications usually end up increasing the risk of more frequent migraines.

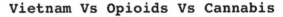

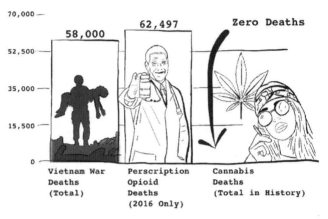

Vietnam Vs Opioids Vs Cannabis

I've seen how quickly opiates such as morphine relieve pain in the most gruesome accidents, but I've also witnessed their destruction. Up to 91 Americans die per day from prescription opioid overdoses.[12] As a result of the doctor-prescribed opioid epidemic, there were more American deaths from drug overdoses in 2016 than deaths in the entire Vietnam war.[13] Zero deaths in history have occurred from any form of cannabis, hemp, or cannabinoids. *(By the way, the graph above shows my tracing skills, which are at about a 3rd-grade level. By the end of this book, my art skills should go up to that of a 5th grader, maybe even junior high.)*

There's a rural town in West Virginia, population 2,900, that prescribed 20.8 million opioid painkillers in the last ten years, which was first reported by Eric Eyre, who won a Pulitzer Prize for his investigative work on opioid "pill mills."[14] Do the math: companies distributing these opioids know they're peddling a legal form of heroin that will cause addiction and abuse.

Prescription opioids are up to 50 times stronger than heroin, which is why drug dealers now mix prescription opioids into heroin. Drug companies and government officials know that a town of a couple thousand people couldn't possibly use all those drugs—20.8 million opioid pills—for medical reasons. Yet some politicians are still more focused on fighting the weed growing in your back yard.

The problem is worsening with failed policies and new synthetic opioids. Deaths from synthetic opioids such as fentanyl have skyrocketed from just a couple thousand deaths in 2012 to over 20,000 deaths in 2016. Researchers from the Centers for Disease Control (CDC) found that people who are addicted to prescription painkillers are 40 times more likely to be addicted to heroin.[15] Prescription opioids are the real "gateway drugs" that are fueling illegal drug deaths.

New studies show that CBD from hemp may reduce opioid cravings and withdrawal symptoms.[16] While opioid deaths were rising across the country, Colorado experienced a 6.5 percent drop in opioid deaths during the two years following legalization of recreational marijuana.[17] Research shows that states that legalize marijuana have a massive dip in opioid use, abuse and overdose rates.[18]

The politicians who say they have no interest in legalizing medical marijuana have no compassion for people living in pain. Once you read about the life-saving effects of cannabinoids on children with drug-resistant epilepsy, with its link to migraine discussed shortly, it will be hard to view any politician who is against medical marijuana as anything but ignorant or inhumane.

You might think that an alternative to pain medications for migraine sufferers is a good thing, as well as curbing the opioid epidemic and saving lives, but there are some pharma bros who don't agree. The opioid maker of a fentanyl spray, Insys Therapeutics, donated $500,000 toward defeating a ballot measure for recreational marijuana in Arizona.[19]

Insys Therapeutics is one tiny pharmaceutical company which succeeded in keeping marijuana out of one state, and you may have heard of them. Insys paid a 1.1-million-dollar fine last year for allegedly bribing doctors to prescribe fentanyl to migraine sufferers and patients with other off-label conditions when it's only intended for cancer treatment.

Drug makers shell out about a quarter of a billion dollars per year for lobbying, making them the largest influencer in politics. You can call it campaign financing, propaganda, wining and dining, legal bribery, or just good old American politics. You can also bet that these large corporations are sabotaging the legalization of marijuana to protect their 11-billion-dollar-per-year opioid market, but they won't win.

According to a recent Gallup poll, 64 percent of Americans, including the majority of Republicans for the first time, support making marijuana legal.[20] Twenty-nine states, plus DC, have legalized marijuana in one way or another and with the sixth largest economy in the world, California, expected to bring in one billion dollars of cannabis tax revenue alone in 2018, the power of money will soon make cannabis legal for pain sufferers across the country.

Fortunately, you don't need to wait for the war on marijuana to end, because you can get legal hemp extract today. There's more to hemp than just pain management. You'll soon learn how hemp attacks the root cause of migraines to prevent migraines from starting in the first place. I'll also break down the best ways to improve hemp's efficacy in fighting migraines. But first, you should understand why this fantastic information is suppressed, because it started long before drug companies wanted to maintain profits.

HEMP HISTORY 101

"There are 100,000 total marijuana smokers in the U.S., and most are Negroes, Hispanics, Filipinos and entertainers. Their Satanic music, jazz and swing result from marijuana use. This marijuana causes white women to seek sexual relations with Negroes, entertainers and any others."

— Harry Anslinger, 1930s

Harry Anslinger was the first commissioner of the Federal Bureau of Narcotics, a predecessor to the DEA, and the federal power behind the illegalization of marijuana.[21] But above all, Harry Anslinger was a fopdoodle, in case you didn't catch that from his quote above. (A "fopdoodle" is an a--hole, which is a word that I will not use here, because fopdoodle is so much more fun.) The bill he sponsored was the Marihuana Tax Act of 1937, which made recreational marijuana illegal.

In the early 20th century the U.S. government renamed cannabis "marijuana" and for unclear reasons spelled it as "marihuana." Many drug policy experts, such as Professor Mark Kleiman of NYU, suggest that referring to cannabis as something that sounded "Mexican" would have made it seem dangerous and would have exploited prejudice against minorities at the time.

For thousands of years, cannabis has been a migraine remedy.

9

In the United States, cannabis was the leading migraine treatment from 1874 until 1942, the year of its removal from the US Pharmacopeia for medical use. Ironically, this was the same year that the U.S. government produced the film "Hemp for Victory," which encouraged farmers to grow hemp to support the production of military uniforms, canvas, rope, and parachutes.

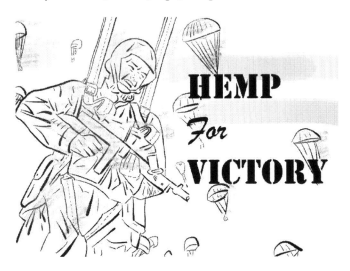

At the time, twelve medical authorities approved cannabis for migraine therapy and protested the ban on medical marijuana.[22] Yes, the irony of governmental support for "Hemp for Victory" combined with the simultaneous illegalization of cannabis as a migraine treatment inspired the title of this book.

Physicians favored cannabis because the alternative was a dangerous drug called ergotamine. Numbness on one side of the body, blue fingers and toes, confusion, and even death are just a few of ergotamine's side effects.[23] Despite cannabis lacking any severe side effects, ergotamine remained the only migraine-specific treatment for the next 50 years. To understand why we discarded cannabinoids from migraine medicine, we need to follow the money.

Lumped under the 1937 Marihuana Tax Act was hemp. The act required farmers to register hemp crops with the Feds and pay unreasonably high taxes. Hemp became much worse than illegal: it was unprofitable. The exception, of course, was during WWII, which was a brief moment of clarity when we acknowledged that hemp was superior to other fibers. When your own life is on the line, you tend to accept logic over profit.

Remember that hemp is a cannabis strain that doesn't get you high because it doesn't contain enough THC. Cannabis illegalization wasn't about protecting people from "reefer madness": it was all about stopping the production of hemp with a sprinkle of racism to fuel the illogical fire.

Shortly after the Marihuana Tax Act passed, in 1938, *Popular Mechanics* magazine published an article titled "The New Billion-Dollar Crop." The authors envisioned a bright future in which hemp would bring jobs to the United States through more efficient manufacturing of paper, fishnets, strong rope, clothing, and thousands of everyday items.

Hemp is ready for harvest in 120 days, as opposed to the 20 plus years it takes trees to grow. An acre of hemp produces up to four times more fiber than an acre of trees and it grows 60 times faster. Hemp fiber is softer and stronger than cotton, doesn't mildew, requires no pesticides or fertilizer, and even replaces petroleum-based plastics. It's environmentally friendly. Hemp paper will last hundreds of years without degrading and can be recycled more times than tree-based paper. Who wouldn't want hemp?

The manufacturing stakeholders at the time already feared the bargain crop that would put a dent in, if not destroy, their more costly way of life. Harry Anslinger may have been the racist face behind reefer madness, but other wealthy fopdoodles didn't like the idea of a hemp revolution either.

William Randolph Hearst was a top financial supporter of the Reefer Madness campaign. Hearst was a timber tycoon and the most powerful newspaper owner in the world.[24] He too was a fopdoodle. (I love that insult: fopdoodle.) Every true pothead knows that Hearst was the guy who said, "Screw hemp. I like being paper rich. We'll create the illusion that marijuana is evil and causes madness, reefer madness, muhahahahhahahaha. That should make all cannabis plants illegal and my trees profitable." Ok, he didn't say all of that, but his actions implied it, which any pothead will tell you.

Andrew Mellon, who was linked by marriage to that federal fopdoodle Anslinger, was the wealthiest fopdoodle on the planet and supported the notion that marijuana evoked rape, murder and violence by "Negroes, Mexicans and Orientals."[25] Mellon was the primary financial backer of DuPont's new synthetic fiber called nylon. In case you didn't know, nylon became kind of a big deal without hemp holding it back. So did plastic, but we won't get into that.

Ok, you get the idea: fopdoodles with money are the reason a powerful migraine treatment became illegal. History repeats itself, again and again. Now it's the pharmaceutical industry that's lobbying against medical marijuana, including hemp, in fear of losing revenue to a new cannabis revolution. Politicians cite our children and crime as the reason for marijuana illegalization, but the raw data doesn't support that claim.

Drug dealers make marijuana accessible to kids because anyone can buy pot off the street as opposed to going into a store and purchasing something that requires a valid identification. Legalizing marijuana replaces drug dealers with regulation, and let's be honest, the war on drugs failed to keep ganja out of our schools. As for crime, prohibition arrests were eliminated when booze became legal. Prohibition's organized crime and the violence that came with those particular illegal operations dried up too.

Reports from the Colorado Department of Public Safety, the FBI Uniform Report, and a comprehensive study from the University of Texas have found that violent crimes have decreased in Colorado, Washington, and Portland, Oregon, after cannabis legalization.[26] Of course, the violence associated with drug dealers self-regulating their market will go down, while arrests from marijuana and the massive cost of incarcerating those arrestees will become non-existent. The billions of dollars in tax revenue could also be used to support programs that detour children from smoking marijuana, or to curb the deadly opioid epidemic with cannabinoids and education, or to improve the lives of residents in legalized-marijuana states however they see fit.

Cannabis has a bizarre history, smeared with groundless

attempts to suppress its medicinal benefits while ignoring the fact that illegalization was all about money. The argument against cannabinoids becomes absurd when we discuss the legal status of non-psychoactive hemp. So, turn the page.

HEMP'S LEGAL STATUS

You can currently buy thousands of hemp products, including hemp extract, online and in retail stores across the United States. Hemp is legal, in a loophole way.

Hemp became illegal to cultivate in the United States under the Controlled Substance Act of 1970. However, you could still import hemp from other countries even though you couldn't grow it here. Even imported hemp that had trace amounts of THC, under 0.3 percent, was deemed legal by a 2004 DEA ruling.[27] This is why you can walk into a store and buy hemp lotion or extract.

More recently, the 2014 Federal Farm Bill allowed for universities and state departments to begin growing hemp right here in the U.S. of A. Since then, 26 states have passed pilot programs for hemp cultivation, which may allow for the commercial production of hemp to study the economics of industrial hemp.[28] Yes, let's examine the "economics" of hemp so that we can help people and bring a lot of tax revenue into our states. Furthermore, according to the Appropriations Act of 2017, federal funds may not be used to prohibit the transportation or sale of hemp grown under the Federal Farm Bill.[29] You can grow it, ship it, and sell it under federal law.

Why do the state and federal government look past the Controlled Substance Act (CSA) of 1970? Because it's a lie. All forms of cannabis, including hemp, were wrongfully labeled as schedule 1 drugs under the CSA. That's the same classification as heroin! You are about to read what a schedule 1 drug is and say, "WTF, is this a joke?"

Drugs must meet two criteria to be labeled as a schedule 1 drug: one, the drug has no medicinal value and two, the substance has a high potential for abuse.[30] It's hypocrisy. The U.S. government has the patent, literally, on cannabinoids for their medicinal use.

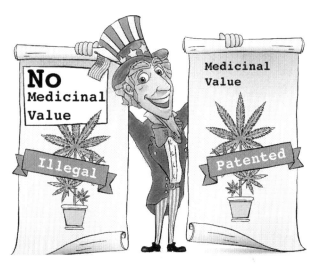

Plus, there are dozens of studies that show cannabis, CBD, and THC have medicinal value. Even cocaine and methamphetamine are not listed as schedule 1 drugs, because they have a limited medical use. Cannabis therefore cannot be a schedule 1 drug.

Law enforcement ignores hemp because it's not psychoactive or addictive and *does* have a medicinal value from CBD. "In humans, CBD exhibits no effects indicative of any abuse or dependence potential," according to robust research from the World Health Organization (WHO). The WHO continues, "several studies have found CBD effective for treating epilepsy and it could be good for a number of other medical conditions."[31] There's only two criteria for schedule 1 drugs and hemp doesn't meet either.

Things get even messier for products labeled as "CBD" or that contain pure CBD. In 2016, the DEA labeled CBD as a schedule 1 drug because it is a "component of marijuana." Luckily, "this action is beyond the DEA's authority," according to Robert Hoban, a professor of law at the University of Denver, "The DEA can only carry out the law, they cannot create it."[32] Furthermore, the DEA has not prosecuted anyone for CBD as a schedule 1 drug because it is not psychoactive or addictive, same as hemp, and the FDA acknowledges 13 states that have legalized CBD for its medicinal value, based on numerous studies.[33]

CBD's legal status has confused authorities because legal hemp extract contains CBD. Hemp companies don't seem too concerned. Pure CBD products are shipped all over the country, with companies claiming that as long as it is derived from hemp, CBD is legal. However, many of the affluent hemp extract companies have removed "CBD" from their product labels to meet federal marketing laws. The word "CBD" is restricted on many advertising platforms (Facebook, T.V., some grocery store chains, etc.), which makes it difficult, but not impossible, to sell. According to Forbes, hemp CBD is rapidly growing in popularity and will become a billion-dollar market in the next three years.[34]

Hemp's manufacturing growth gives consumers confidence because the federal government won't prosecute an individual customer while it allows manufacturers to produce millions of dollars' worth of hemp extract. Even state lawmakers are turning on the federal government to get rid of this ridiculous classification of hemp and CBD. California state lawmakers recently passed a resolution that calls on Congress to reschedule all forms of cannabis, including hemp, CBD, THC, and other cannabinoids, so that cannabis can be sold and studied for its known medical benefits.[35]

Hemp is given added protection under state cannabis laws. A federal court ruling in 2016 stated that the DEA could not expend resources to interfere with state medical marijuana laws.[36] Even Congress' latest budget bill under the Trump administration, at the time of this writing, says that "none of the funds available to the Department of Justice may be used to combat state medical marijuana laws."[37]

Allen Peake is a Georgia lawmaker, conservative, and Christian, and he is defiantly challenging the federal government. Georgia's medical marijuana laws do not allow for the cultivation of cannabis, nor do federal regulations allow for cannabis to be cultivated or imported to Georgia. So, what does a good American do for people in need? State representative Peake "donates" $100,000 of his own money every year to cannabis research in another state, he then "magically" receives a box of cannabis oil on his state desk, he does not ask how it got there, and he then distributes it to patients as gifts.[38]

Why would Allen Peake blatantly risk federal drug trafficking charges? There are children with intractable epilepsy, meaning medications don't work for them, who have experienced a complete or significant reduction in seizures from CBD-rich cannabis.[39] Allen Peake refuses to turn these patients away, or other patients with chronic conditions. The federal government looks the other way because they know the law is baseless and what kind of monster would tell parents that they can't have life-saving cannabis oil for their child with epilepsy?

If a state representative is publicly challenging state and federal cannabis laws, there is little chance that the government will attack consumers of non-psychoactive hemp. Now that half of U.S. states are relying on cannabis taxes, remaining states will probably pass laws to legalize cannabis too. Most people expected Republicans to continue to support illegalization, but that didn't appear to happen in Congress's latest budget, and that's not expected to change now that illegalization will mean the loss of funding for critical state programs, like education.

Things are changing. Nevada state officials declared a state of emergency for a marijuana shortage, shortly after recreational marijuana became legal in the state. We are talking about a conservative state where possession of a single marijuana cigarette was a felony and resulted in up to six years in prison, a longer sentence than the average rapist serves. The difference now: politicians do not want to lose those tax dollars and will do whatever it takes to keep cannabis products selling.

With the progress of medical marijuana laws, hemp may become completely legal without relying on legal loopholes. There are currently several bills awaiting Congress' vote, which specify that hemp and CBD are not schedule 1 controlled substances because they are not.[40]

Hemp has a bright future. The Federal Farm Bill and the Appropriations Act of 2017 give us the ability to purchase hemp and restrict the federal government from interfering legally. You can continue to buy hemp extract with about the same risk as purchasing hemp soap at your grocery store, which you've been able to do since the 1970's. However, things could change and you want to stay up to date on the laws.

Part II: Migraine and Hemp

WHY HEMP HEALS MIGRAINE

To understand how hemp can heal migraines, we need to know why migraines happen in the first place. The official cause of migraine is unknown, but we know a lot about what triggers migraines. A migraine trigger is what I call a "migraine key," because it can turn migraines on or off.

A few of the most common migraine keys that trigger migraines are MSG, aspartame, nitrites, glutamate, dehydration, stress, pollution, weather, and allergens. The removal of migraine triggers and the things that prevent those triggers from inducing migraines are also migraine keys. If dehydration were a migraine key that turns migraines on, water and electrolytes would be the migraine keys to turn migraines off.

Battling migraines is straightforward if you know what your migraine keys are, but if you don't, it's like trying to open up a door that has several locks, while you are fumbling around with several hundred unmarked keys. Finding your triggers is the hard part, especially if a migraine monster is chasing you, because migraine triggers are individualized and unique. Painstakingly unique, with no known commonality between them. Until now.

A study published by the American Headache Society in December of 2015 evaluated all the major migraine triggers and found a distinct correlation.[41] The study concluded that this relationship was likely the unifying principle behind nearly all migraine triggers. The authors came to the same conclusion that I did in my first book, which was published in the same month after I systematically evaluated all the major migraine triggers: migraines are a defensive mechanism of the human body.

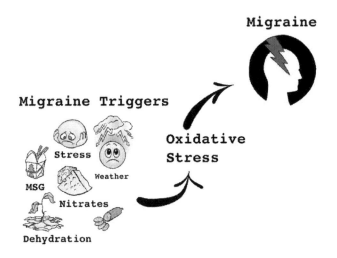

The common thread between all migraine triggers is called oxidative stress. High levels of oxidative stress are associated with a four-fold increase in the risk of migraines.[42] Migraine triggers raise levels of oxidative stress, and migraine sufferers are more likely to have high levels of oxidative stress.

If migraines are indeed a defense mechanism against something deadly, we would see tons of diseases with higher levels of oxidative stress and migraines. So, do we? Do we find conditions that hurt the human body associated with higher levels of oxidative stress and migraine prevalence? Yes.

There are over forty conditions that increase the risk of migraine. Heart attack and stroke, epilepsy, multiple sclerosis, hypothyroidism, IBS, anxiety, obesity, and fibromyalgia are just a few. Search on Google or PubMed for any of these conditions combined with the term "oxidative stress" and you will be floored by the results: oxidative stress is the common denominator. I have compiled the research for you, with links to all the studies, in an article titled "Forty Conditions Associated with Migraine" at migrainekey.com.

Oxidative stress is a universal migraine key. This is the beginning of an answer, a solution. This answer explains the links between all the migraine research that I evaluated in my first book. I found that all common migraine triggers were associated with inflammation. Inflammation is a result of oxidative stress. So oxidative stress is the underlying problem, an underlying problem that has solutions.

You may not know what oxidative stress is, but it's likely you know what antioxidants are. If oxidative stress is the universal migraine key that turns all migraines on, antioxidants would be the universal migraine key that turns all migraines off. However, it's not as simple as the food industry makes it sound. You are not going to cure migraine with a blueberry muffin that contains "antioxidants."

Antioxidants are more of a process than something located in your blueberry muffin, according to research published by Harvard.[43] We need to go back to junior high school science. Bear with me. I live for this nerd stuff and you should too because it is the answer to migraines, health, happiness, and feeling all-around good. This process also explains why hemp may change your life.

Free Radical

Normal

Oxidative Stress

Oxidative stress occurs when a molecule loses an electron and turns into a free radical. Free radicals arise from things that hurt the human body. Remember free radicals from your junior high science class? Those are the lonely electrons circling a molecule and it hurts to be lonely. Electrons are supposed to be orbiting the nucleus in pairs, not alone. These lonely guys are damaged goods and as soon as they see a healthy molecule with a happy electron-pair couple dancing around, the lonely guys get radical. The free radical says, "give me your partner" and then steals one of the electrons from the healthy molecule.

The problem is, you can't just steal someone's partner and soul mate. That will lead to problems in your home. The first molecule remains damaged. Not only that, the once-healthy molecule that just lost a happy electron becomes damaged too, another free radical, and it goes on to steal another molecule's electron and the process continues. The process spirals out of control until all the molecules are damaged goods and the entire cell dies. That, my friend, is oxidative stress.

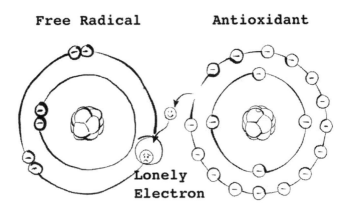

An antioxidant stops this downward spiral. An antioxidant sees the first lonely molecule and donates an electron to that molecule. Antioxidants break the chain reaction that ultimately leads to cellular death. It's a process.

There are a lot of antioxidant foods that help, but most of the processed foods that list antioxidants on the package do not increase antioxidants in your body. For example, a blueberry muffin is going to provide some antioxidants that donate electrons, but the inflammatory sugar in that muffin will ultimately cause more oxidative stress than it reduces.

Let's say you have a neurological disorder, like migraine or epilepsy. Most antioxidants only have a limited capacity to make it to the brain and throughout the body. Eating a couple of blueberries might not have enough antioxidant power to make it into the trillions of neuron synapses in the brain. There are many different antioxidants, with different roles, that all play a unique part in lowering total oxidative stress in the brain and body.

The preliminary research on cannabinoids shows that they have the antioxidant capacity to make it to the brain and reduce total levels of oxidative stress with neuroprotective qualities.[44] [45] [46] A growing number of studies prove that CBD has antioxidant abilities.[47] The antioxidant properties of both THC and CBD would explain why medical marijuana reduces migraine frequency and pain.

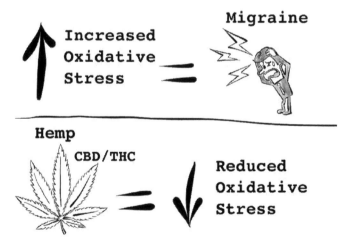

The universal migraine trigger, oxidative stress, is the reason most drugs fail migraine sufferers. Triptans can stop migraines, possibly by their acute ability to constrict blood vessels and raise a happy chemical in the brain called serotonin. With every up, there is a down. The happy chemicals may not stick around, but the side effects do. Triptans cause side effects that end up raising levels of oxidative stress in the body.[48] If too many triptans cause oxidative stress, wouldn't that mean more migraines?

A study published by the Institute of Neurology, Italy, found higher levels of oxidative stress in chronic migraine sufferers who overused either anti-inflammatory drugs or triptans.[49] In theory, anti-inflammatories should reduce oxidative stress. However, the study found medications decreased antioxidant capacity of chronic migraine sufferers, which increased oxidative stress and thus migraines.

Any drug that is overused or causes severe side effects will harm the body. Things that hurt the body produce oxidative stress. In the end, the medication becomes less efficient, people, in turn, use more medicine, the side effects cause more oxidative stress, and migraine frequency ultimately goes up.

Unlike migraine medications, CBD in hemp may go straight to the root problem and reduce oxidative stress. Antioxidants are the reason CBD may reduce migraine, while oxidative stress is the reason most medications end up making migraines worse.

HEMP IS NOT A MEDICAL "CURE"

Hemp is not a medical cure for migraines; there is none. A medical cure eliminates a disease, kills it, there's no coming back. Migraines are a defensive mechanism for the body and may return with exposure to high levels of oxidative stress.

The American Diabetes Association says essentially the same thing about type 2 diabetes. A medical cure isn't possible because diabetes is a natural response to excessive glucose and will come back if the patient is exposed to things that trigger that natural reaction.

You are looking for the type of "cure" we use in everyday language, the definition you'd find in a standard dictionary: to restore health. The layman definition of "cure" is not only possible to achieve but proven by a plethora of studies.[50] Research shows that migraines can be eliminated in as little as three days.

Successful migraine studies have accomplished complete migraine remission by adjusting the headache threshold. The headache threshold is like a cup. We add headache triggers to the cup and eventually they spill over, triggering a headache or migraine. Reducing the top triggers can prevent the threshold from ever overflowing.

A study published in 1983 removed significant food triggers from participants' diets and found that non-food triggers, like stress, became dormant and did not affect migraines after starting the diet. Eighty-nine percent of patients became migraine free, which is a higher success rate than any medication ever developed. (Don't worry, I'll detail the best food eliminations and other ways to eliminate migraines in addition to hemp later). This perplexed scientists: how could unrelated headache triggers become dormant?

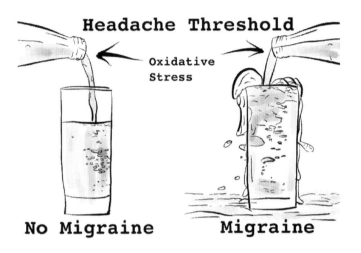

You know why. Migraine triggers share a commonality. The cup is filling up with oxidative stress and removing large amounts of oxidative stress from any part of the body may prevent the threshold from overflowing. That is the reason why a diet change or using hemp can reduce or eliminate migraines that are caused by multiple triggers. You are merely taking volume out of the cup, so it doesn't overflow.

Diets that reduce oxidative stress and migraines suggest that migraine is the world's most advanced health-monitoring system. There are over forty conditions associated with migraine, they all come with oxidative stress, and migraines are a defense mechanism for that oxidative stress. Genetics play a role, but only when oxidative stress is present.

MIGRAINE GENETICS

Migraine genetics can remain dormant for most of your life until a trigger brings the beast to life. A case study published in 2002 found that a man developed migraines for the first time at the age of 57 after introducing soy supplements to his diet.[51] Soy allergies are a common migraine trigger. Allergens increase oxidative stress. After the removal of soy from his diet, voilà, symptoms completely disappeared. This case study, among many others, challenges the idea that migraines are permanent and irremovable.

Migraine is a system that's more common than you would think. Up to 43 percent of women will experience migraines at some point in their lifetimes.[52] However, only when triggers are present do migraines appear. Over 18 percent of American women experience migraines on a regular basis and about one billion people worldwide suffer from migraines.

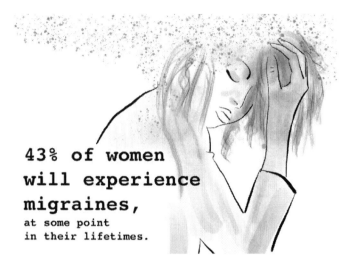

43% of women will experience migraines, at some point in their lifetimes.

Migraines are far too prevalent to serve no purpose. Pharmaceutical companies love to tell you, "just keep taking the drugs, there is no migraine cure, it's genetic, nothing you can do about it." They want you to feel helpless and drug dependent. Genetics make you susceptible to migraines but are not the cause of migraine. That would be comparable to saying, "heart disease is genetic and there's no way to prevent it." Of course, you can prevent preventable diseases that have genetic predispositions.

A diet study published in the *Lancet* in 1979 was a breakthrough in migraine treatment. The elimination diet eliminated migraines in 85 percent of patients and all patients drastically reduced their migraine frequency. Most patients were migraine free in three days. Stop and think about how amazing that is. Similar results were replicated in the 1983 study, mentioned earlier, and later in a 2007 migraine elimination-diet study.[53] Genetics only trigger migraines when oxidative stress hits the top of the threshold, which research proves.

A study published in 2017 by the European College of Neuropsychopharmacology—what a mouthful—studied migraines and a gene that regulates stress and sleep.[54] There was no link between migraines and this gene. They found nothing unusual until they looked at participants who experienced financial hardship and stress. Bam, the gene that regulates stress and sleep was associated with migraine when a significant migraine trigger that affects both stress and sleep was present. Sleep deprivation and psychological stress cause oxidative stress and increase the risk of migraines, and death. The genetics of migraine sufferers are smart enough to warn the body of this deadly buildup.

It sounds overdramatic, and it is. You are not going to die from one bad night's sleep. Your body will take care of that little bit of oxidative stress tomorrow, don't stress. But years of inadequate sleep and stress take a toll. I was well aware of this, waking up in the middle of the night to the sound of an alarm, paranoid that somewhere someone needed help because they did. The broken sleep pattern and stress of a firefighter are associated with an increased risk of heart attacks, which are promoted by oxidative stress. Those firefighters don't just get heart attacks because of their genes; something triggers it.

You know what can help your genes with sleep and stress? Hemp. And we'll go in-depth on how hemp helps with sleep and stress in the section on stress. Another fantastic way to improve your sleep schedule is by setting an alarm clock, but not just for the morning, set an alarm clock one hour before your bedtime. When you hear the alarm go off, disengage from all activities that keep you awake, like looking at electronic screens, and get ready for bed. A sleep schedule can do wonders for overall health and migraines, as is noted in multiple studies. Your genetics might make it difficult for you to sleep, but that's only more reason to adamantly help your body overcome migraine genetics.

Urban Africa is the best example of migraine genetics in action. Rural Ethiopia has a migraine prevalence of about three percent, which is consistent with most of rural Africa, but studies show that their neighbors living in urban conditions have six to ten percent of the population living with migraines.[55] The same International Headache Society criteria for migraine was used to compare rural and urban neighbors because doctors often misdiagnose migraine. Not just in Africa, the misdiagnosis rate of migraine in western countries, such as the United States, is around 50 percent, according to the National Headache Foundation.[56] But with only four hours of headache education, who's to blame?

The same genetics only produce migraines when exposed to headache triggers. In Ethiopia's case, urban headache triggers. Genetics can't be the cause of migraines if genetically similar neighbors have double or triple the migraine rates.

Rural people have many health advantages, such as adequate sunlight, good posture, organic food, social support, and exercise. They aren't exposed to hundreds of food chemicals while sitting in a cubicle all day. The lack of modern-day luxuries put rural people at a lower risk of the top preventable diseases and a substantially lower migraine risk.

Over 38 genes are identified as susceptible to migraines. Some genes make people more sensitive to migraines than others, but only when there is prolonged exposure to migraine triggers that hurt the human body.

Genetics may increase the risk of migraines and oxidative stress, but that doesn't mean we can't use natural methods of reducing oxidative stress and migraines, like hemp. We can't all live like rural Ethiopians, but we can try to remove some of our triggers and get a little help from hemp along the way.

Why use hemp if you can just remove the headache triggers that trigger migraines? Diet, health, genetics, food triggers, and other migraine triggers are individualized and often difficult to discover. Hemp can help reduce oxidative stress while you are figuring out your unique triggers.

In some cases, migraine triggers can't be removed or managed with diet alone. For example, a neck injury will raise oxidative stress levels and may not have a quick fix. In this case, hemp could help reduce oxidative stress, inflammation and pain in hopes of reducing or eliminating migraines.

There are multiple conditions associated with migraine. We don't have all the answers for preventing something like fibromyalgia—wide-spread muscle pain and fatigue—which is associated with migraines and oxidative stress. If fibromyalgia triggers migraines, CBD may help reduce its symptoms. In fact, fibromyalgia and migraine patients reported some of the highest levels of relief from CBD-rich cannabis in an extensive survey completed by the medical marijuana industry in California.[57] All patients (100%) with migraines and fibromyalgia reported a decrease in pain, which is unheard of for even the most potent opioids.

CBD may help control oxidative stress from a neck injury or fibromyalgia, but we can't ignore other common triggers of oxidative stress. They all fill up the headache threshold and you should acknowledge them while benefiting from hemp.

Hemp is not guaranteed to work, nothing is. However, new and stunning cannabinoid research suggests that hemp is going to help a lot of migraine sufferers. For some, cannabinoids may reduce oxidative stress levels to a point where migraine genetics and the majority of migraine triggers are no longer an issue.

CANNABINOID-MIGRAINE RESEARCH

The First Medical-Marijuana-Migraine Study

The first migraine clinical trial for cannabis was published in May of 2016 by the University of Colorado, Anschutz Medical Campus.[58] Since 1942, universities have shunned cannabis research because of the illegal nature of marijuana. When I say shunned, I mean the researcher would go straight to jail, without collecting $200. Cannabis is still federally illegal. We're lucky that the University of Colorado doesn't give a flying fig about federal law.

The result of the Colorado study was nothing short of phenomenal. The study included 121 migraine sufferers who used various forms of cannabis, including vaporized, smoked, edible and topical cream.

The average dose per month per participant was 2.64 ounces for vaporized or 1.59 ounces for smoked cannabis, which might be comparable to your neighbor who was high last night, high this morning, high before lunch… basically high all the time. 1.59 ounces for a monthly cannabis dose works out to more than four joints per day.

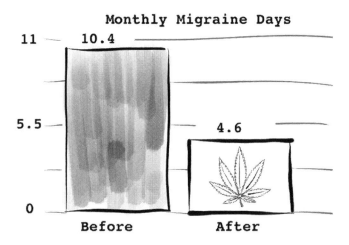

Monthly Migraine Days

The results: migraine frequency decreased from a group average of 10.4 migraine days per month to 4.6 migraine days per month. Eight-five percent of migraine sufferers reported a decrease in migraines. Impressive results, dare I say, *high marks*.

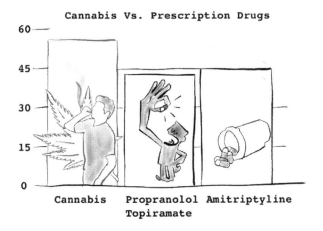

Cannabis Vs. Prescription Drugs

There was a 56 percent reduction in total migraines for the total group. To give you an idea of how this compares to the top migraine prevention drugs, propranolol is at 43 percent, topiramate is at 43 percent, and amitriptyline is at 45 percent for total migraine reduction in a total group. [59] [60]

What medication statistics don't tell you is that migraine prevention drugs usually have serious side effects that will increase oxidative stress, making the drugs less useful over time. Migraine studies don't typically last beyond three months, partially because of cost, and because over time the efficacy of migraine drugs dwindle down while side effects ramp up.

The average use of medical marijuana in this study was 22 months, a substantial amount of time. Twenty-two months is enough time for a patient to find that the migraine reduction is not just a placebo effect and in fact, the marijuana is working. It's also enough time for patients to be like, "I've been high for so long that I don't remember what it is like to not be high. This is more fun than migraines."

The study wasn't perfect, with inconsistent cannabis doses and strains, and no placebo group. However, this inconsistency also makes the research impressive.

Strains high in CBD are reported by migraine sufferers to be more effective. Some of the migraine sufferers in this study probably used marijuana with low CBD and high levels of pesticides and mold. That'll hurt the body and decrease effectiveness.

Doses too high in THC could increase oxidative stress and as you can imagine, many marijuana strains have been hybridized for the last century with the goal of having more THC, to get you stoned, man. Inhaling the smoke form of cannabis is undoubtedly unhealthy and will also add a level of oxidative stress.

A consistent dose of a cannabis strain that is recommended for migraine sufferers and administered healthily is almost guaranteed to improve the results of this study. But that doesn't address the pink elephant in the room. Bills, kids, work, and blah, blah, blah, means that you can't just go down to the lake and be high, all day, every day. Or at least many people can't.

Cannabis strains that are low in THC, or ultra-low in THC like hemp, will be more tolerable to migraine sufferers who can't afford the psychoactive effects of typical marijuana strains. High CBD and low THC cannabis may be even more effective than this study, especially after using methods that increase the medicinal strength of CBD.

This book is focused on hemp, but there are also ways to use medical marijuana products that will not get you high. One way is called micro-dosing. Micro-dosing is when you take THC dosages that are too small to have psychoactive side effects. This is essentially what a full-spectrum hemp extract provides.

Hemp extracts vary. They can have a CBD to THC ratio of 20:1, 25:1, 30:1, or no THC at all. So, for example, at a 30:1 ratio you take a dose of hemp extract that contains 30 mg of CBD and you get 1 mg of THC with it. However, micro-dosing usually refers to taking a small enough dose of a medical marijuana product that it does not get you high, usually having under 2.5 mg of THC. We'll get to this in more detail when we discuss dosages in a later chapter.

When people say, "I tried marijuana and it made me high, paranoid, and lethargic, and then I freaked the heck out," they are talking about an overdose, not a treatment. If you took a bunch of migraine prevention drugs without following a doctor's prescription, you would also be in trouble. There are many cannabis strains with varying quantities of cannabinoids, so overdosing on a single strain doesn't mean that you can't succeed with low doses of a CBD-rich cannabis strain.

Migraine in Rats

A 2018 study published by researchers from Washington State University found that THC eliminated migraine-like pain in rats when given in the right dose and in a timely manner.[61] Waiting 90 minutes or using a dosage too high or too low did not work, similar to what you'd expect from other migraine drugs.

The pain test measured the rats' ability to run on a wheel, which as you can imagine, gets to be questionable for rats that are too stoned. The rats that were administered high doses of THC gave up running, probably because high rats just want to lay around and eat a bag of chips. However, the wheel running test is still a useful way to assess this migraine treatment, because "only treatments without disruptive side effects will restore normal activity," according to the study.

The need to "restore normal activity" is one more reason to consider micro-dosing THC. Disruptive side effects such as being uncontrollably giggly or unable to function in society are indicative of THC doses that are too high. On a serious note, side effects may generate oxidative stress and increase migraine risk. High-dosage THC is better for acute migraine relief and a day spent in bed as opposed to a day in the office. Consistently high levels of THC for more extended periods of time may do more harm than good.

The researchers—from the above 2018 study—proved that THC delivers anti-migraine effects by stimulating the CB1 receptor, but does not entirely reverse a migraine as noted by anecdotal human reports on cannabis use. (You'll learn more about the amazing CB1 receptor soon.) But THC is not cannabis. The researchers tested THC alone and indicated that using additional cannabinoids may abolish migraines, as opposed to just providing stupendous pain relief. Let's look at what a mix of CBD and THC does to humans.

A New Cannabinoid-Migraine Study

A new study presented at the Congress of the European Academy of Neurology found that cannabinoids were just as effective as amitriptyline, a leading migraine prescription drug.[62]

The research team, led by Dr. Maria Nicolodi, administered the combination of 18 mg of CBD and 38 mg of THC per day to 79 chronic migraine sufferers. After three months, the CBD/THC combination produced slightly better results than amitriptyline: another cannabinoid win. However, the cannabinoids also reduced the pain intensity of migraines by 43.5 percent and that is terrific news.

Migraine medications are either for prevention or acute relief, not both. Cannabinoids have the rare ability to prevent migraines and reduce the pain of migraines once they hit.

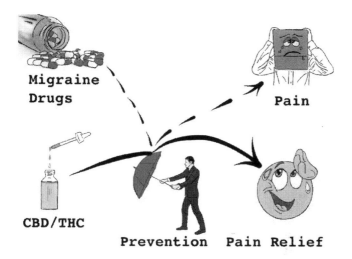

The researchers also found that inflammation in the gut, aka irritable bowel syndrome, which is common in migraine sufferers, decreased in patients. Most migraine medications increase gut problems. Reducing inflammation in the second brain—the second brain is the gut, which I'll elaborate more on later—is a necessary component of long-term migraine prevention. The CBD/THC combo seems to be different from migraine medications in all the right ways.

There are a few takeaways and considerations from the new research. Doses of less than 9 mg of CBD and 19 mg of THC per day produced no effects during initial testing. 18 mg of CBD per day is very doable. Some migraine sufferers are using five times as much CBD per day (100 mg) as used in this study, while others benefit from just 5 mg of CBD per day.

38 mg of THC per day is a lot, in my opinion. That much THC will get the average Joe dreadfully high. I tried a gummy bear once that had 5 mg of THC, the lowest dose, and I was high as a kite. I have a very low tolerance for cannabis and THC. I would not be able to work after taking a 38 mg dose of THC because I'd probably be too entertained by heightened vision and sounds, and maybe leprechauns, while many other people would do just fine.

CBD counteracts the "high" effects of THC, but drowsiness

and difficulty concentrating were still side effects in the study. However, the side effects were considered minimal and "highly positive" by the researchers, in comparison to migraine medications.

The study only used THC and CBD, missing out on other cannabinoids, vitamins, minerals, and terpenes from natural hemp that increase the chance of reducing migraines. This study, like the prior, may benefit from using more CBD and less THC.

Cannabinoid-and-Migraine Research Takeaway

The takeaway from the initial cannabinoid research is that CBD has a real potential to beat conventional migraine medication. Before you go out and buy some CBD, you should know how cannabinoids affect a natural system in your body that is "one of the most important physiologic systems involved in establishing and maintaining human health," according to research published in 2013 by the University of Maryland School of Medicine.[63] It's called the endocannabinoid system. Its relation to migraines is captivating. You are about to read my favorite chapter, and Sondra's favorite chapter too—Sondra, you remember, my wonderful wife, who no longer gets migraines.

THE EXTRAORDINARY
ENDOCANNABINOID SYSTEM

A new theory published in a 2016 study states that an endocannabinoid deficiency may be the origin of migraine.[64] The research team was led by none other than Dr. Mechoulam, the godfather of cannabinoids. Let's work our way forward from the 1960s to understand how plausible this new migraine theory is.

An Israeli scientist, by the name of Dr. Raphael Mechoulam, identified the first cannabinoid, THC, in 1964. CBD was discovered soon after.[65] "By using a plant that has been around for thousands of years, we discovered a new physiological system of immense importance," Dr. Mechoulam recalled.

Scientists followed the cannabinoid pathways in the late 1980s and early 1990s and discovered that cannabinoids bind to at least two receptors, appropriately named cannabinoid receptor 1 (CB1) and cannabinoid receptor 2 (CB2).

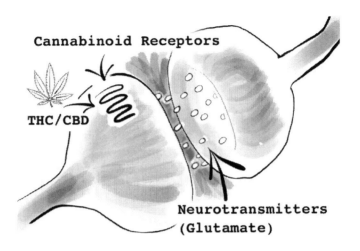

But why do we have these cannabinoid receptors in the first place? What purpose do they serve, besides getting you high?

How the endocannabinoid system affects human health is the focus of Dr. Mechoulam's life's work. In 1992, Mechoulam and a team of researchers discovered that smoking ganja was not the only way to activate the cannabinoid receptors. Our bodies make their very own cannabinoids called endocannabinoids, "endo" meaning "from within." Mechoulam named the first endocannabinoid "anandamide," after the Sanskrit word for bliss.

Anandamide plays a core role in the feelings of motivation and pleasure. Anandamide helps produce the sense of "runner's high," which is just as much of a mechanism of biological survival as it is a feeling of happiness.[66] The discovery of anandamide opened Pandora's box. It was the first of many endocannabinoids discovered which began to unravel a prehistoric system that regulates human health: the endocannabinoid system.

Have you ever run into a high guy who said, "This is my medicine, man," as he finished a joint? His musk would linger with a woody smell, maybe Palo Santo. I always thought that guy, there's one in every town, was just high. It turns out he was talking about the enormous role that the endocannabinoid system plays in the biological functions of human existence. And to think you scoffed at him.

The endocannabinoid system is responsible for maintaining homeostasis. Dr. Mechoulam wasn't kidding around when he said "a system of immense importance." Homeostasis is the ability of the body to maintain equilibrium or stability internally when faced with changes externally. That means everything you think it does.

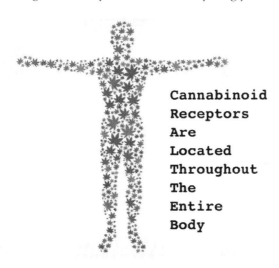

Cannabinoid Receptors Are Located Throughout The Entire Body

Cannabinoid receptors are located throughout the entire body and control the immune system, inflammation, energy production, appetite, memory, nutrient transport, stress response, anxiety, the autonomic nervous system, temperature, blood pressure, sleep, and more.[67] In other words, endocannabinoids balance your health.

Every positive influence that cannabinoids have over migraine is the result of the balancing act of the endocannabinoid system. For example, if too much glutamate is sent between the synapses in the brain, blocking the neurotransmitter pathway, it can trigger a migraine or seizure. This destructive process is called excitotoxicity. It excites cells to death and results in oxidative stress.[68]

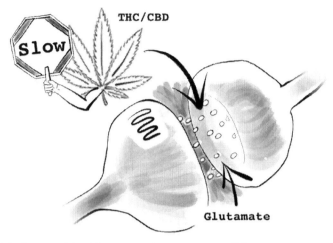

THC/CBD

Slow

Glutamate

Endocannabinoids are the most well-known retrograde messengers, and possibly the only retrograde neurotransmitters, which retroactively send messages back to an overactive nerve, saying, "Slow down, dude, you are sending too much glutamate too fast."[69] Endocannabinoids are like your own little cannabis doctor telling your brain that you are overexcited, chill out, slow down, and here is a chill pill before you excite yourself to death. Have you heard a cannabis doctor speak? That's how they sound.

Because overactive nerves, excitotoxicity, and oxidative stress are involved in neurodegeneration, the endocannabinoid system is under research aimed at preventing oxidative-stress-related conditions, from stroke and traumatic brain injuries to Alzheimer's and Parkinson's disease, migraine, and many more.[70]

According to the medical authority Medscape, "modulation of the endocannabinoid system may be a cure for chronic neurologic and immune conditions." Migraine is a neurological condition, but a study recently published in the journal *Nature Genetics* suggested that migraine could also be an immune system disease.[71] If an endocannabinoid deficiency exists in migraine, immune system function is also likely to go out-of-whack, because endocannabinoids help control the immune system in addition to neurological health.

One night last week, I started to get a bad cold and I took 15 mg of hemp extract. By morning, I was a little tired, but all my symptoms of the cold were gone. Vanished. Yeah, I'm one guy, writing a book on hemp, claiming that hemp cured my common cold. Sure, I've never had this happen before, but I acknowledge it could be a placebo effect. However, research shows that cannabinoids can fight off infections with anti-inflammatory activity and can even significantly reduce the replication of powerful viruses such as hepatitis C.[72] [73]

All you need to do is look at the vast list of auto-immune conditions associated with migraine (e.g., fibromyalgia, lupus, multiple sclerosis, etc.) to realize that a healthy immune system is essential for fighting migraines.

So, the big question is, does an endocannabinoid system deficiency exist in migraine patients? I'm glad you finally asked, you smart cookie you.

A 2008 study published in the journal *Neurobiology of Disease* found that chronic migraineurs had an endocannabinoid system that functioned at only 50 percent compared to the endocannabinoid function of healthy individuals.[74] You can imagine that a system of "immense importance" is going to wreak havoc on the human body if it's only functioning at 50 percent. Your cannabis doc would be like, "I'm giving your endocannabinoid system a grade of F-, dude, your body is out of order."

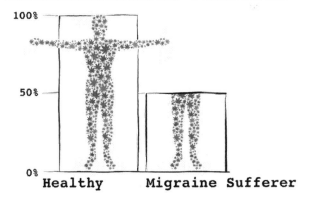

Endocannabinoid Function

You can also bet that the catastrophic problems occurring within the endocannabinoid system didn't happen overnight. They must have progressed for a long time before the entire system plummeted to half speed. Multiple studies now support this theory, with findings of reduced endocannabinoid levels in the cerebrospinal fluid of migraine sufferers, and endocannabinoid dysfunction in related conditions.[75]

Fibromyalgia and irritable bowel syndrome (IBS) are two of the most common comorbidities of migraine, and guess what: they are also associated with endocannabinoid deficiency. Most notable about these conditions is that traditional medicine— prescription medication—provides a level of treatment that is pathetic. The drugs are far from adequate.

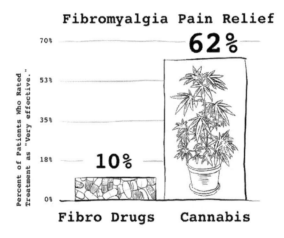

In the 2016 National Pain Report over 60 percent of fibromyalgia patients said prescription medications "do not help at all." Only ten percent of patients listed medications as "very effective."[76] Cannabis provides the opposite level of relief, in a good way, with 62 percent of patients claiming cannabis is "very effective" and only five percent saying that it "does not help at all." It's no shock that cannabinoids help with conditions that are related to endocannabinoid deficiencies.

How do we know cannabinoids will help with endocannabinoid deficiency? You ask an important question. Cannabinoids bind to the endocannabinoid receptors and produce the same effects. However, it also appears that cannabinoids will help improve the function of the endocannabinoids we already have.

New research found that CBD alleviated the psychotic symptoms of schizophrenic patients as effectively as prescription medications.[77] The study, published in the journal *Translational Psychiatry*, attributed the alleviation of schizophrenia symptoms (anxiety, depression, hallucinations, etc.) to a measurable rise in anandamide signaling or the "bliss" endocannabinoid. This surge of endocannabinoids is one of many examples that prove that the cannabinoids from external sources can help your internal endocannabinoid system.

If endocannabinoids are so important to human health, what would happen if we took them away? If you were an evil drug company, you could try that, on real people. A pharmaceutical company tested out a drug called Rimonabant to see what would happen if they blocked endocannabinoids from binding to CB1 or CB2. Cannabinoids control appetite, so why not block the cannabinoid receptors of thousands of obese people?

The idea of a magic pill that eliminates appetite is alluring. Blocking an entire system that we know very little about is appalling. Rimonabant was being tested to reduce the risk of cardiovascular disease in obese folks but marketed as a weight-loss drug, which after 33 months failed to show any significant improvement in patients.[78] Rimonabant did, however, significantly increase gastrointestinal, neuropsychiatric, and fatal psychiatric side effects. Four patients committed suicide and the trial abruptly ended.

Four dead people. Four dead people with families and pets and friends. Let's focus on improving the endocannabinoid system and not blocking or destroying it. The side effects of a weak functioning endocannabinoid system will be vast and this, of course, brings us to oxidative stress.

Endocannabinoid Deficiency, Oxidative Stress, and Migraine

At this point, you may be wondering if it's oxidative stress or endocannabinoid dysfunction that causes migraine. First, I will say that the official cause of migraine is unknown. Migraine is the most sophisticated defense mechanism, alerted from numerous complex conditions and headache triggers that harm the body, and is more advanced than all of our progress in science combined. That said, what we do know about oxidative stress, endocannabinoids, and migraine is fascinating.

It's clear that an endocannabinoid deficiency will create oxidative stress if the body loses homeostasis. If the endocannabinoid system goes rogue, you won't be able to control glutamate, energy production, stress, or any other factors that trigger migraines.

On the other hand, we know that a ton of conditions and nearly all migraine triggers are associated with oxidative stress. Vast amounts of migraine research imply that oxidative stress is the initial culprit. Is there only one "cause" of migraine or are these systems connected?

What is oxidative stress in its simplest terms? Oxidative stress is caused by just about any external force that harms the human body. The endocannabinoid system maintains homeostasis or stability internally when faced with changes externally. Oxidative stress disrupts homeostasis. The endocannabinoid system controls homeostasis. It's yin and yang.

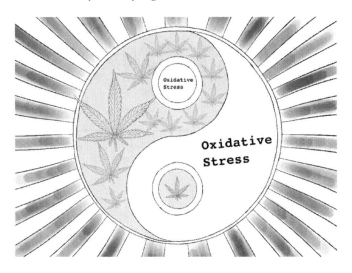

Yin and yang are not just negative and positive, light and dark, but two forces which are complementary to each other. You can't have one without the other. (Just think of me as Sensei Jeremy for the next few paragraphs.) The endocannabinoid system controls homeostasis. Homeostasis is maintained by controlling oxidative stress with an antioxidant process called redox, short for the reduction of oxidation.

The processes of oxidative stress and reduction of oxidation happen simultaneously and neither can occur independently, according to *The Gale Encyclopedia of Science*. The endocannabinoid system is therefore connected to oxidative stress every step of the way. One does not exist without the other. If oxidative stress sounds confusing, that's because it is, and when you figure it out, you should let scientists know, because they may be able to cure virtually every disease from understanding the exact pathway of oxidative stress.

The concept of something hurting and healing the body at the same time is confusing. It is happening now as you breathe. Every breath of oxygen you take in is turned into energy and left oxidized. This small amount of oxidative stress is no problem because homeostasis controls it with an antioxidant process. It happens simultaneously. Just make sure your body has what it needs to produce enough antioxidants and endocannabinoids.

New research confirms that the endocannabinoid system has a direct connection to oxidative stress. Lab rats were injected with toxins at the University of Bialystok, in Poland. The response was a reduction of antioxidants and an increase in oxidative stress and endocannabinoid activity.[79] Something hurts the body, antioxidants are depleted, oxidative stress occurs, and the endocannabinoid system is activated to maintain the equilibrium that we call life.

Growing evidence suggests that these two systems "cross-talk" to maintain homeostasis: "Whereas abnormalities in either system may propagate and undermine the stability of both systems, thereby contributing to various pathologies associated with their dysregulation," according to research published by the University of Dundee, Scotland, in April of 2016.[80] That is a profound statement for migraine sufferers, but right now I'm thinking, "Does the University of Dundee have anything to do with Crocodile Dundee, and whatever happened to that guy?"

It's like this: a healthy endocannabinoid system is needed to control oxidative stress and the control of oxidative stress is required for a healthy endocannabinoid system. Problems in the endocannabinoid system lead to issues with oxidative stress and vice versa. Yin and yang.

What does this mean for migraine sufferers? Migraine sufferers should be aware of all the triggers that increase oxidative stress, all the methods that increase antioxidants, and all the measures that improve the endocannabinoid system. We are dealing with one system that is interconnected.

As we move forward, the endocannabinoid system will explain how hemp heals migraines and at the same time, we will discuss how to improve those results by decreasing oxidative stress and increasing antioxidants. But first, you now have sufficient evidence to buy some hemp, if you haven't already. Let's jump into the different options of cannabinoids and the best ways to use them.

Part III: Guide to Buying Hemp

EVERYTHING YOU NEED TO KNOW ABOUT BUYING HEMP IS HERE

FAKE HEMP

A fugazy is old Italian slang for counterfeit products—think of a fake diamond purchased off the street. You should have the same mindset as a mobster when purchasing hemp because, like buying a diamond from the black market, there are no rules or regulations. A mobster has an advantage over you, or at least myself, when purchasing a fugazy because he or she is scary and will probably demand a couple of fingers along with a refund, plus interest, of course. I would just hope that no one notices my shiny new cubic zirconia, living the rest of my life as a lie.

According to a 2017 study published in the journal *Epilepsy and Behavior*, the FDA investigated CBD products and found that most contained little-to-no CBD.[81]

Only two out of 24 products tested had the amount of CBD on the label. The rest had either no CBD or only trace amounts of CBD, while others contained high levels of THC.

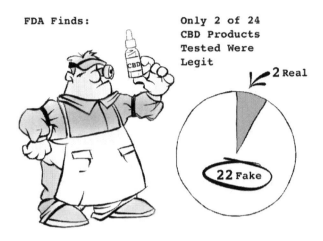

FDA Finds: Only 2 of 24 CBD Products Tested Were Legit

2 Real

22 Fake

These companies are vile. Many people use CBD as a last resort for painful neurological conditions; the last thing they need is to waste money on a lie. Since we can't go after these companies with violence, we must use the more respectable gangster tactic of making sure the product is tested before we buy, thus eliminating the risk of purchasing a fugazy. You don't want to risk buying fake hemp extract and then give up on something that could have changed your life.

In the FDA study, they neglected to test the largest CBD manufacturers, which makes me think the FDA was attempting to find unethical companies, as they should. A recent study, published in the journal *JAMA*, tested 84 CBD products from 31 companies and found that nearly 70 percent were mislabeled, however 42 percent actually had more CBD than specified, while others contained less CBD or substances not listed on the label.[82]

Look for reputable companies that use third-party testing. They're out there. Some companies will even send every batch of extract produced to an independent testing facility to ensure that their product is consistent with their claims. Independent labs also test for high levels of impurities such as lead or other natural toxins found in virtually all produce.

Produce typically contains levels of lead and other metals that are too low to be harmful to the human body. Don't be too worried about vegetables. There are low levels of metals in natural soil, water, livestock, and in you right now. It's everywhere and not a problem in small doses. However, metals and other toxins can be a problem when consumed in high doses.

Because hemp grows like a weed, it absorbs a lot more toxins than say, an apple. Toxins from natural metals or unnatural pesticides may cause oxidative stress and harm the endocannabinoid system. Good manufacturing processes and testing can avoid this.

You need a cannabinoid product that is tested for the nutrients you want and tested for the toxins you don't want. Don't go cheap, because if it's fake, what's the point?

THE ENTOURAGE EFFECT

The entourage effect coupled with minimal side effects make hemp extract the best cannabinoid option for the majority of migraine sufferers, hands down. Neither pure CBD nor pure THC come with the entourage effect.

Both THC and CBD have a sweet spot for medicinal benefits known as the bell-shaped response. Like any medication, if you take in too little, it doesn't work, if you absorb too much, it doesn't work.

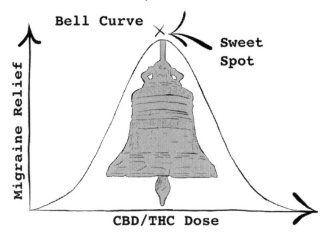

THC and CBD are known for activating the cannabinoid receptors to reduce oxidative stress and inflammation, but they can also block the cannabinoid receptors and have the opposite effect.[83] [84] "It seems to be a dose-dependent issue," according to a review of cannabinoid research published in 2016.[85] Taking too much CBD or THC may increase oxidative stress and therefore dampen migraine relief or even trigger migraines. Dun dun duuuun!!!

You never want to hit the top of the bell-shaped curve. The top of the bell-shaped curve is like that moment when you realize that your last sip of coffee took you from energetic to jittery. It is the shot of liquor that took you over the top, one pot-brownie too many, an overdose. The top of the bell-shaped curve is when feeling good becomes overpowered by side effects and oxidative stress.

This is where the entourage effect steps in. **The entourage effect is what researchers refer to as the synergy of multiple nutrients found within the hemp plant that increase medicinal benefits, counter side effects, and maintain benefits at high doses.** Highlight that last statement, because the part about "multiple nutrients found within the hemp plant that increase medicinal benefits" may change the treatment of migraines and many other diseases in the near future. But before we get to that, let's discuss how the entourage effect avoids the bell-shaped curve by preventing oxidative stress and side effects.

I may have scared you with the research that states that too much CBD can induce oxidative stress. However, the doses of CBD used in research, which we'll get to, are extremely high and even at those high doses CBD comes with little-to-no side effects. THC, however, is a concern. THC is a pink-elephant-in-the-room type of concern.

Let's say that you took a dose of isolated THC and it provided migraine relief. Then, you got wild, and took another dose of pure THC, but instead of more migraine relief, your body slides down the back side of that bell-shaped curve. Rather than feeling good, you feel the inflammation, anxiety, paranoia, mental sluggishness and psychoactive effects that high doses of isolated THC can bring.

CBD has you covered. CBD is not the only cannabinoid that is part of the entourage effect, but it is the most well studied. CBD is proven to reduce the side effects of THC in multiple studies.[86] I researched this last statement, I wrote about it, I thought about it deeply and I was still surprised by the feedback I recently received from a friend whom I gave a bottle of hemp extract to. He used 25 mg doses of hemp extract to completely control his anxiety at work, but that didn't surprise me, and it won't surprise you after reading the chapter on stress.

What did surprise me is that he said he smoked cannabis after taking the hemp extract and it completely eliminated the anxiety and mental sluggishness that he experienced from cannabis in the past. His experience startled me. What if the majority of people who have had a negative experience from the medicinal use of cannabis were simply overdosing on THC and lacking CBD? What if his experience with the entourage effect was common?

Small doses of THC can increase the happy brain chemical called serotonin, but high doses can reduce serotonin levels.[87] It's possible that low serotonin from too much THC was causing my friend's cannabis-induced anxiety, which the entourage effect from hemp completely reversed. Low serotonin is also a migraine trigger. I would bet that CBD-rich cannabis—or taking CBD-rich hemp with cannabis—would help migraine sufferers who previously found cannabis useless. Of course, there is research to back up my bets.

Indiana University researchers in September of 2017 gave adolescent and adult mice either high doses of THC or high doses of THC with CBD.[88] The mice given pure THC experienced increased anxiety and impaired memory, while the group given THC with CBD had no undesirable effects. This is synergy at its finest.

A 2010 study published in the journal *Pain Symptom Management* found that terminal-cancer patients who experienced no pain relief from opioids also found no measurable relief from isolated THC.[89] However, cancer patients absorbing both THC and CBD experienced a 30 percent drop in what was a previously untreatable pain. This CBD/THC synergy of increased medicinal benefit and reduced side effects has also been witnessed in multiple animal studies.

The entourage effect is about so much more than combining THC and CBD. The entourage effect research is saying: Isolated cannabinoids don't perform as well as the entire cannabis plant. We have solid evidence that CBD improves the medicinal benefits of THC, but there are other compounds in cannabis that may combine with both THC and CBD to increase their medicinal value.

Hemp extracts can contain over 80 different cannabinoids, including CBC, CBG, THCV, CBDV, CBN, and many others. These cannabinoids are not as well studied, but initial research is impressive and shows these additional cannabinoids may improve the entourage effect for migraine sufferers.

Lesser-Known Cannabinoids:

CBC

CBC stimulates the endocannabinoid system and has shown anti-inflammatory, pain-relief, antibiotic, and antifungal properties during initial animal testing.[90] It also reduces THC intoxication in mice, which is what synergy is all about: creating a balance.

CBG

CBG is the next most effective cannabinoid against breast cancer after CBD, surpasses THC in pain relief, and regulates serotonin, suggesting it may be an antidepressant. Breast cancer is not as likely in migraine sufferers for unknown reasons, according to a 2016 study of over 160,000 people, but hey, it's still good to avoid.[91] An antidepressant with pain relief is a plus for migraine relief.

THCV

THCV promotes energy and weight loss in obese mice, which is the opposite effect of THC. A small study in humans found that THCV reduced the side effects of THC.[92] Go, synergy.

THCV also has anti-seizure, anti-inflammatory, and antioxidant properties, which relieve symptoms in animal models of Parkinson's disease.[93] Stage two clinical trials are currently underway by GW Pharma for the use of THCV in type II diabetes treatment, and THCV has potential for treating epilepsy and autism disorders too.

Parkinson's disease and epilepsy are linked to migraine. There are many clinical similarities between autism and migraines and anecdotal evidence suggests autistic patients are more likely to have migraines.[94] THCV sounds like it should be tested on migraine sufferers next.

CBDV

CBDV is a close relative to CBD, although less studied, and a precursor to THCV, so it's likely to add to the same positive effects on the endocannabinoid system. CBDV shows anti-seizure effects in animals and is currently under trials for treating epilepsy in humans.[95] Migraine sufferers need some CBDV in their lives.

CBN

CBN is a byproduct of THC and amplifies its sedative effects, which promote a better night's sleep.[96] It has anti-seizure and anti-inflammatory properties. CBN inhibits breast cancer cells, although only in large concentrations.

CBN stimulates stem cells in bone marrow for bone health, which may prove useful for migraine sufferers. The endocannabinoid system protects against bone loss, which is why cannabinoids, including THC and CBD, are under research for treating osteoporosis.[97]

Osteoporosis is bone destruction that is associated with and may be caused by oxidative stress.[98] So, endocannabinoids protect bone health and oxidative stress destroys bone health. What's that mean for migraine sufferers, who are more likely to have oxidative stress and a weak endocannabinoid system?

A study of more than 80,000 people found that the risk of migraines is tripled in osteoporosis patients.[99]

The endocannabinoid system and the possibility of it treating migraines continues to impress you. It does, right? Yeah, yeah it does.

Cannabinoids Combined Are Amazing

The combined research on these individual cannabinoids suggests that using a hemp extract with multiple cannabinoids will increase the medicinal benefits of both THC and CBD. There are also dozens of other cannabinoids that we know nothing about and I can't wait to see what they will do for migraine sufferers.

Terpenes may be just as beneficial for migraine prevention and the entourage effect.

Terpenes

At the base of essential oils and cannabis are terpenes. Ask any group of migraine sufferers if essential oils ease migraines and you will find that many sufferers swear by them. Terpenes are used in aromatherapy and, in addition to their well-studied medicinal benefits, emit aromas of citrus, earthy, spice, peppermint, and 200 other flavors. Terpenes are the reason why cannabis strains have distinctive smells like bubble gum, lucky charms, or skunk.

Some of the terpenes found in hemp are myrcene, beta-caryophyllene, linalool, pinene, nerolidol, bergamotene, limonene, and alpha-humulene. Each terpene helps the endocannabinoid system prevent migraines in their own unique ways.

I know that you might be thinking, "essential oils have no place in modern medicine and are reserved for hippies who base medical care on 'feelings.'" Well, you are at least partially wrong because the hard research on terpenes is about to knock your socks off.

β-Caryophyllene

β-Caryophyllene is the most abundant terpene found in cannabis strains and may also be the most impressive. Its anti-inflammatory effects are on par with indomethacin, a potent drug occasionally used for migraine. However, indomethacin should not be used for migraine because of its gastric side effects, which may increase migraines in the long run. Unlike indomethacin, β-Caryophyllene protects the gut instead of destroying it.[100]

β-Caryophyllene protects the brain against oxidative stress in diabetic rats, Parkinson-disease-model rats, and rats with metabolic dysfunction.[101] [102] Migraine has a link to glucose problems, Parkinson's disease, and metabolic (energy production) problems. The antioxidant power of β-Caryophyllene should make you consider a full-spectrum hemp extract over isolated CBD or THC alone.

Linalool

Linalool provides the soothing anesthetic effects found in lavender, which are equal to the strength of menthol. Linalool may be the reason that lavender is a favorite essential oil for migraine relief, especially for soothing the nerves in the face and neck. Migraine sufferers love menthol too. Linalool slows down the migraine trigger glutamate and reduces nerve pain and seizure activity. It also decreased the need for morphine in patients that underwent surgery in a study published by the New York University Medical Center.[103] Morphine-level pain relief for migraine? Yes, please.

Pinene

Pinene treats inflammation in the lungs and expands oxygen flow, which is a good thing for migraine prevention. Inflammation in the lungs from asthma or allergens dramatically increases the risk of migraines. Pinene's best synergistic role in the endocannabinoid system is improving memory, which may counteract the side effects of THC.[104] Go, go, go, synergy.

Myrcene

Myrcene is best known for triggering the "couch-lock" phenomenon when combined with THC. Myrcene is a natural muscle relaxer and may leave you unable to get off the couch if mixed with large amounts of THC.[105] Relaxing muscles in the neck and face may take pressure off the nerves associated with migraine. Also, myrcene protects against stroke and heart attack by reducing oxidative stress.[106] Over 20 years of research has found that migraine increases the risk of cardiovascular disease by 50 percent.[107] Yeah, migraine sufferers want relaxed muscles, without heart attacks.

Nerolidol

Nerolidol is a component in orange peels that may prevent migraines by protecting against excitotoxicity and oxidative stress, although it is best known for treating fungal growth and reducing tumors in rats.[108] [109] You don't want migraines or tumors or fungal growth.

Limonene

Limonene neutralizes gastric acid and supports the gut.[110] It is used for heartburn, gastric reflux, weight loss, lung inflammation, and prevents several types of cancer.[111] Improving the gut, lungs, and metabolism will aid migraine prevention from multiple angles. Oh, we'll get to how vital the gut is for migraine relief in a later chapter.

Bergamotene

Bergamotene is one of the terpenes in sweet basil that may be responsible for basil's antioxidant and anti-inflammatory properties.[112] Yep, those attributes should attack migraines too.

Humulene

Humulene is found to reduce inflammation on the skin and in the airways.[113] [114] It may also reduce skin inflammation such as acne with antibacterial properties.[115] Children with migraine have seven times the odds of having acne, which is predictable because acne is linked to inflammation and oxidative stress.[116] Oxidative stress "may be an early event that drives the acne process," according to research published by the SUNY Downstate Medical Center in New York.[117]

How can we bottle this stuff? Get rid of migraines and acne with humulene.

Terpene Synergy

You know when you read the side effects of a drug box and think, "could this be any worse for me?" I feel like we just read the opposite list and right now I'm thinking, "hemp is the best medicine ever created."

There are so many medicinal benefits of cannabinoids and terpenes that we can't possibly know what specifically in cannabis reduces oxidative stress and migraines. The entourage effect presents the same conundrum we face with vegetables: we know that certain whole vegetables, such as broccoli, reduce oxidative stress, but taking isolated vitamins with the same amount of antioxidants does not produce the same results.

Synergy is accepting the measurable health effects of something in its natural whole form, even if its components do not provide the same results individually. Oh, but we're not finished with the entourage effect yet.

Omega-3 and Omega-6 Fats

Researchers from the University of Nottingham, United Kingdom, found that healthy fats can significantly improve the absorption of cannabinoids into the body. Essential fatty acids administered to rats in addition to cannabinoids increased the amount of CBD in the blood by three-fold.[118]

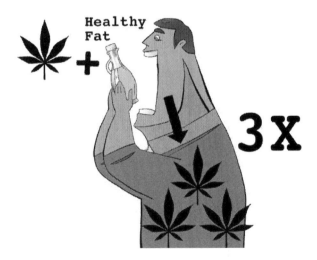

You get up to three times as many cannabinoids inside the body by adding healthy fats to the cannabinoids you take in from outside the body. And we know that cannabinoids convert to endocannabinoids once inside the body, which is how CBD fights migraines. CBD is like a fat-soluble vitamin, the absorption rate skyrockets when the body has healthy fats available.

Fortunately, you don't need to slurp a spoon full of butter with your CBD because many hemp extracts naturally contain omega-3 and omega-6 fatty acids. Additionally, some hemp extracts mix in hemp seed oil, which provides even more healthy fats. This isn't to say your consumption of healthy fats should end with hemp extract.

There is a whole lot of research that shows that diets that are rich in healthy fats and low in carbohydrates are a good thing. How good? We will discuss the incredible success rates of fats and ketones for migraine sufferers in the upcoming section on healthy fats. For now, consider a quality hemp extract with natural fats included.

Hemp Minerals

Hemp extracts may include trace minerals such as iron, calcium, magnesium, and potassium. Research shows that iron helps prevent menstrual migraines, or migraines during that time of the month, which is common in most female migraineurs.[119] Calcium, magnesium, and potassium are electrolytes required for hydration and migraine prevention.

The trace levels of these minerals in hemp extract won't cure anyone's migraines, but they could help a bit. We'll discuss all the minerals you need for migraine prevention in the upcoming section on hydration and hemp.

Hemp Vitamins

Hemp contains low levels of vitamins B1, B2, B6, and D.

B Vitamins in Migraine Success

Vitamin B2 became famous as a migraine treatment after it cut the migraine days of patients in half during a study conducted by Humboldt University of Berlin, Germany.[120] If this study was done by Humboldt State University, located in the "marijuana region" of California, the results might have been higher. I'll explain what cannabinoids plus B vitamins do for migraine prevention in a hot second or however long it takes you to read the next couple paragraphs.

B Vitamins Reduce Homocysteine and Migraines

A 2009 study published from Griffith University, Gold Coast, Australia, found that vitamins B6, B9, and B12 successfully reduced homocysteine levels, which are elevated in migraine sufferers, and cut migraine disability in half.[121] The study put B vitamins right up there with top-notch migraine medications and it's likely due to this reduction of homocysteine, because homocysteine induces oxidative stress.

Endocannabinoids and Homocysteine

You know that if reducing homocysteine is a good thing for migraine prevention, endocannabinoids must also play a role here. Indeed, anandamide protects against homocysteine and oxidative stress.[122] Anandamide was described earlier as the "bliss endocannabinoid," which is increased by the absorption of CBD. B vitamins seem to share the same goals as endocannabinoids: reduce homocysteine, reduce oxidative stress, and reduce migraines.

B9 Increases Endocannabinoids

What if we combine endocannabinoids and B vitamins? Let me answer the above question with the title of a study published in the *European Journal of Pharmacology*, "Stoners eat your broccoli: Folic acid enhances the effects of cannabinoids at behavioral, cellular, and transcription levels." The title, and that is the real title of the study, says it all. Vitamin B9 increases the absorption of anandamide and THC in lab rats by up to 129 percent.[123]

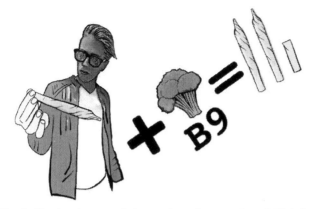

That's like buying one joint and getting another 1.29 joints for free. What a bargain. (Just in case you were wondering why there are candles in the picture above: those are joints and don't you dare make fun of my artistic joint-rolling skills.)

Now, we don't know if the absorption rate of endocannabinoids and cannabinoids in humans will be so dramatic, but this study lets us know that endocannabinoids and vitamin B9 somehow work together and feed off each other's success. Let's consider using both B vitamins and endocannabinoids to reduce oxidative stress and migraines.

Methylation

It's critical to note that the low levels of B vitamins found in hemp will not supply enough of all the B vitamins you need. B vitamins are part of a process which helps the body create energy and reduce toxins and oxidative stress. Sound familiar? Endocannabinoids regulate energy, toxins, and oxidative stress. Endocannabinoids are part of this complicated process, called methylation, but we still have a lot to learn about exactly how endocannabinoids spin the methylation process.[124]

Vitamin B2, B3, B6, B9, and B12 are necessary B vitamins for the methylation process to reduce oxidative stress and migraines. That's why B vitamins are beloved by migraine sufferers.

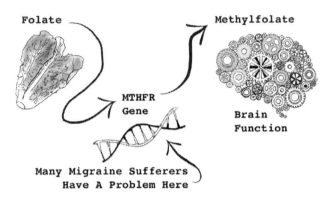

Folate + MTHFR GENE = Methylfolate

The MTHFR Gene

Many migraine sufferers have a mutation in the MTHFR gene that reduces the body's ability to convert folate (vitamin B9) into methylfolate. Folate from leafy greens doesn't make it into the brain without this conversion. The process that creates methylfolate is called methylation and because many migraine sufferers have a genetic problem here, they either need to supplement methylfolate or ensure that they are consuming lots of folate from leafy greens and other vegetables. *(I'd like to point out that if I had known how long it would take to trace a brain made out of gears—image above—I never would have started this masterpiece. Each little gear represents time that I'll never get back, ever. Ever!)*

Methylation is Complicated

This process gets confusing fast. At the end of this section, I'll provide info about my article on the subject, which contains an animated video on the process and also links to a video from the leading MTHFR expert. The critical thing to remember is that endocannabinoids and B vitamins work together in the methylation process to reduce homocysteine and oxidative stress, which will reduce your migraine risk.

Because endocannabinoids may use methylfolate in the fight against migraines, and the fact you may already have low levels of methylfolate to begin with, you want to make sure you obtain enough methylfolate, as well as other B vitamins.

The B Vitamin Answer

According to a leading MTHFR gene expert, Dr. Benjamin Lynch, taking both the premium versions of vitamin B9, called methylfolate, and vitamin B12, called methylcobalamin, may reduce the problem that the MTHFR genetic predisposition brings. Therefore, methylfolate and methylcobalamin should reduce the risk of migraines.

The supplement manufacturer "Seeking Health" makes "B Complex Plus," which has all the premium B vitamins included or you can take a quick dissolve vitamin B9 and B12 called "Active B12 with L-5-MTHF." By the way, this supplement gives me energy and I feel great after taking it.*

> *I have no affiliation with any supplements. Take at your own risk. Only buy from a trusted source, because, as the New York Times reported, supplements are not FDA regulated and often contain substances not on the label or are entirely fake.[125]

Of course, an abundance of natural foods is the best way to get all the B vitamins, but supplementation is helping a large percentage of migraine sufferers.

B Vitamin Summary

Endocannabinoids and B vitamins work together to fight migraines. Hemp contains low levels of vitamins B1, B2, and B6. Make sure you have enough of all the B vitamins by eating leafy greens and other vegetables and/or consider a supplement of the premium B vitamins.

For more on this fascinating subject I recommend reading my article on migrainekey.com titled "Migraine Prevention: B Vitamins" and visiting Dr. Benjamin Lynch's website at

MTHFR.net to learn more about the MTHFR genes linked to migraine (MTHFR C677T and MTHFR A1298C).

Vitamin D

Vitamin D is found in hemp and is needed to produce the happy brain chemical called serotonin.[126] Vitamin D is why you feel so glad after getting a little sunshine. Vitamin D deficiencies are associated with oxidative stress and migraines. Anything that reduces oxidative stress will benefit the endocannabinoid system. There's also some preliminary evidence that suggests a direct link between vitamin D and healthy endocannabinoid function.[127]

These low levels of vitamins in hemp might not help. You can get more vitamin D from walking out into the sun for five minutes. However, it is possible that these vitamins in combination may help the synergy of hemp just a tad bit.

The Entourage Effect Summed Up

The entourage effect increases the medicinal benefits of CBD and THC, all while reducing the side effects. It may be from terpenes, other cannabinoids, healthy fats, or the low levels of other nutrients found in the hemp plant. Give your cannabinoids the best chance for fighting migraines by purchasing a hemp extract that has the entourage effect. There are a few things you'll want to look out for when purchasing the perfect bottle of hemp, which I'll go over in the next chapter.

WHAT TO LOOK FOR IN A HEMP EXTRACT

The best hemp extract is one that contains CBD, other cannabinoids, vitamins, minerals, and terpenes. It must come from a reputable company that tests for purity and impurity, and you should look at multiple review sources online that vouch for their product. The hemp extract should come from leaves and flowers, sometimes referred to as "aerial parts," of CBD-rich hemp. For example, hemp seed oil does not contain CBD and you need to look for "hemp extract." Keep in mind that hemp seed oil may be added to "hemp extract" to improve absorption.

Because "CBD" is restricted from many marketing platforms (e.g., Facebook, television, supermarkets, etc.), many manufacturers do not list CBD on the label. "Phytochemicals," "phytonutrients," or "full spectrum" are often mentioned instead of CBD. Many products will only list the milligrams (mg) on the front of the bottle, which is typically the amount of CBD or cannabinoids in the product. Check with the manufacturer and ask for a third-party test of the level of cannabinoids in their product.

If you are in a state where medical marijuana is legal, you may want to consider a cannabis extract with high levels of THC and CBD. I recommend hemp extract instead because it avoids the potential side effects from THC. The little bit of THC in certified hemp goes a long way.

"THC has twenty times the anti-inflammatory potency of aspirin and twice that of hydrocortisone," according to a peer-reviewed study published in 2008.[128]

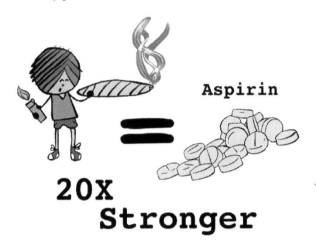

It's possible to benefit from THC, even if you don't get high, similar to how people take pain medications for pain while others take a whole bunch of pain meds to get sloshed. If you feel exceptional from cannabis extract with high levels of THC, go for it. You can also try micro-dosing, which we'll get to.

I get this question a lot: "What brand should I buy? Just tell me the perfect hemp extract or cannabis strain to get." There is not enough clinical evidence to recommend a particular brand or strain of hemp or cannabis for migraine. The cannabinoid profile, terpenes, and other nutrients may have a unique effect on each individual. It's also hard to say which is the best when there isn't enough research on the lesser known cannabinoids and terpenes that add to the entourage effect.

Cannabis strains fall in the same boat. We know we want a strain that has high concentrations of CBD, but beyond that, it's unknown which of the hundreds of strains is best for migraine. It's like trying to compare if raspberries are healthier than blackberries or blueberries. They have different nutrients that could be equally healthy.

Legalization of medical marijuana will help researchers provide answers to these questions in the future. Cannabis companies are also collecting data on which strains people prefer with any given condition. It's also likely that once a cannabis strain is found best suited for the average migraine sufferer, growers will be able to use hybridization to bring the THC down to a level as close as possible to hemp without lessening the medical benefit for migraine.

I researched the hemp market for about six months while consulting with a cannabis company that wanted to create and conduct a study on a hemp extract designed explicitly for migraine sufferers. The astronomical cost of doing a study and the limitations imposed by the FDA on marketing such a product led to the cannabis company deciding not to pursue the project for now. However, after speaking with dozens of manufacturers, I did find two reliable companies that sell hemp products which may benefit migraine sufferers. (Though neither company makes any medical claims about their products.) Both companies' products provide the full entourage effect mixed with healthy fats for increased absorption.

Currently, at the time of this writing, the two most reputable hemp extract companies, in my opinion, are Bluebird Botanicals and Charlotte's Web. Bluebird Botanicals does multiple third-party tests on their cannabinoid profile, which they proudly post on their website. Each product has a batch number on it, so you can see the third-party tests of exactly what's in your hemp. They also have excellent customer service. Bluebird is the best deal for an authentic product and that's where my wife and I currently get our hemp extract, for now at least.

Charlotte's Web is the most well-known hemp extract company. Their hemp helped treat a little girl named Charlotte's epilepsy, and her case study became famous, which we'll discuss soon. Charlotte's Web is more expensive than Bluebird and provides lower levels of CBD, but slightly higher levels of other cannabinoids. They also have phenomenal customer support. Charlotte's Web is on the front lines of the push for federal legalization of hemp and CBD. They are funding the legal battle that will hopefully make hemp extract recognized for its medicinal use.

Whether these reliable companies are the best choice for migraine is unknown because there just isn't any migraine research on specific hemp extracts. I would also caution that the reputation of a company and how they do business can change overnight. I'll try to keep an updated list of reliable hemp products at migrainekey.com, but you should always do your own research as well.

BEST WAYS TO ABSORB CANNABINOIDS

There are several ways to absorb CBD: inhalation, oral, sublingual, or topical cream. Each form of hemp has its own benefits and drawbacks, which makes each application useful for particular situations. There are times, such as during a migraine day, that you may choose to use all four methods. The following is a bare necessities guide on how to take cannabinoids for migraine.

Inhalation

Inhaling CBD is the fastest way to increase CBD in the blood, taking only a couple of minutes for the body to fully absorb. If there's one thing that pharmaceutical companies know about migraines, it's that time is of the essence when attempting to abort an approaching migraine. This is why the famous Excedrin Migraine has added caffeine, to speed the delivery of the drug into the blood. They even make injectable versions of triptans, just to shave a few minutes off absorption time.

In the need for speed, inhaling CBD is the best approach to take when you first recognize a migraine coming. Vaping can also immediately reduce stress, the most common migraine trigger.

The drawback of CBD inhalation is that it provides the shortest amount of relief time, approximately one-to-three hours.[129] CBD immediately rises to high levels in the blood, and steadily leaves the body over a four-hour period. Most vape juice is from CBD isolate, which is missing other cannabinoids, terpenes, vitamins, healthy fats, and other nutrients which may increase the medicinal benefits of CBD. Accurate dosing can also be a problem. However, new vape products are coming out—such as "Dose Pen" by the company Dosist—that measure each dose, are third-party tested, and provide multiple cannabinoids and terpenes.

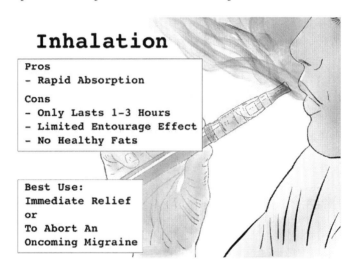

Inhalation

Pros
- Rapid Absorption

Cons
- Only Lasts 1-3 Hours
- Limited Entourage Effect
- No Healthy Fats

Best Use:
Immediate Relief
or
To Abort An
Oncoming Migraine

The short burst of CBD makes inhalation great for aborting migraines, but not ideal for preventing migraines, because it typically lacks the full entourage effect and does not provide stable levels of CBD throughout the day. We need more research on inhaling any type of vapor from these new devices, but you should absolutely avoid vape juice with artificial additives that may damage your lungs, and purchase a product with natural ingredients. CBD vape juice also doesn't have enough research to recommend it at the high doses necessary for long-term migraine prevention. You can, however, inhale CBD when you need to and use other forms of CBD for daily migraine prevention.

Oral

Oral administration is swallowing a pill of a full-spectrum hemp extract with all of its cannabinoids, terpenes, vitamins, and nutrients. It provides the most gradual release of cannabinoids into your system, which lasts for about seven hours. You get the fats, which triple the absorption rate and the synergy of all the other nutrients. All of this comes without the awkwardness of smoking a vape or the unpleasant taste of a liquid extract.

There are also options of taking pure CBD isolate, often mixed with coconut oil, for those who prefer high doses of pure CBD. Just make sure that the CBD isolate is pure and tested for no additional chemicals, used during extraction, which may contribute to more gut inflammation.

The downside is that pills last the longest, but also take the longest to absorb: about 30 to 90 minutes.[130] Since pills are absorbed through the gut, which is often inflamed in migraine sufferers, this may not be a good option for all migraine sufferers. The milligrams of CBD in each pill is also set (e.g., 25 mg) and not adjustable. This makes it hard for a migraine sufferer to find his or her optimal CBD dosage because she or he is most likely taking too much or too little.

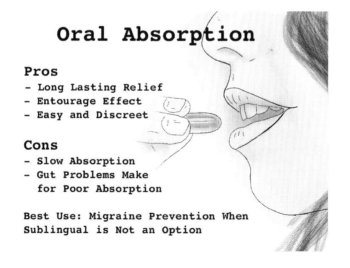

Oral Absorption

Pros
- Long Lasting Relief
- Entourage Effect
- Easy and Discreet

Cons
- Slow Absorption
- Gut Problems Make
  for Poor Absorption

Best Use: Migraine Prevention When
Sublingual is Not an Option

The pills can come in handy for those who don't like the taste of hemp extract and have found a CBD dose that works for them. It's the easiest and most socially acceptable way to take CBD discreetly.

Oral absorption also applies to edibles, which are more common of medical marijuana products. Edibles add an extra degree of uncertainty to the dosage and ingredients of a product because manufacturers often test cannabinoid profiles before mixing the extract into a batch of cookies, brownies, chocolates, candy, or whatever. "Whoops, I added a thimble too much, no big deal," thought the guy making your ganja cookie. But dosage, cooking, and storage make a difference in the final cannabinoid profile and its migraine prevention abilities. For these reasons, a pill or extract is a better choice for a consistent dose of migraine prevention.

Sublingual

Hemp extract can be absorbed sublingually by placing the liquid drops under the tongue for 30 to 90 seconds before swallowing the remainder of the liquid. Sublingual absorption begins within a minute or two, the blood has high levels within 15 minutes, and peak levels are found in the blood in about an hour.[131] Sublingual administration bypasses the gut and rapidly absorbs CBD through capillaries in the cheek and under the tongue.

Swallowing the remainder of the extract allows the body to absorb the rest of the cannabinoids and nutrients slowly. As with the pills, hemp extracts that contain healthy fats may increase absorption by up to three times.

The downside is that a natural hemp extract contains terpenes, which are healthy but make it taste earthy. There is no beating around the bush here: hemp extract doesn't taste good. The first time I tried it, like most people, I said, "It doesn't taste great, but it's tolerable." I like natural products and will put health above taste and as I said, it's not that bad.

Some companies mask the flavor, slightly, by adding chemicals, artificial flavors, and natural flavors. Of course, artificial flavors are top migraine triggers, but natural flavors can be just as bad. Natural flavors are chemicals that are extracted and mixed in laboratories into hundreds of different formulas. Many natural flavors contain excitotoxins such as free glutamic acid, which includes the same chemical compounds that make MSG a top migraine trigger. Excitotoxins, such as aspartame, free glutamic acid, or MSG, may excite cells to death and trigger migraines.

Avoid natural and artificial flavors if you can. To be fair, some natural flavors are entirely healthy and the small doses of other chemicals found in a flavored hemp extract may be too low to trigger a migraine, but it's something to consider. And if the flavor is too good to be true, you might want to make sure the product does, in fact, contain hemp extract.

There are companies that sell CBD isolate with no other cannabinoids, THC, terpenes, or other nutrients. Because CBD has no flavor in itself, taste is not an issue with CBD isolate. This is an excellent choice for someone who cannot have THC or requires ultra-high doses of CBD. The CBD isolate is usually mixed with a healthy fat such as hemp oil, olive oil, coconut oil, or MCT so that the body can adequately and safely absorb it sublingually or orally. You may hear the company refer to the added oil as a "carrier oil."

The extraction process of quality hemp is expensive. CBD isolate is cheaper and faster to manufacture because they don't need to preserve all the other nutrients. They can also use low-quality plants because all the nutrients are filtered out anyway. However, the likelihood of fake CBD isolate products is higher because it doesn't have a distinctive taste, so you should be extra careful that a third party tests the product. I spoke to one of the largest cannabis product distributors in California, who shall go unnamed, and he suspected that most of the CBD products in cannabis dispensaries, such as CBD water or CBD gummy bears, don't contain any CBD.

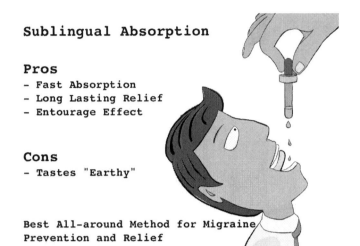

Sublingual Absorption

Pros
- Fast Absorption
- Long Lasting Relief
- Entourage Effect

Cons
- Tastes "Earthy"

Best All-around Method for Migraine
Prevention and Relief

Sublingual administration is the best all-around method for taking cannabinoids. It absorbs fast, can provide a full spectrum of nutrients for the entourage effect, lasts almost as long as the pill form, bypasses the gut, and it is easy to adjust the dosage. You can start off with a few drops and work your way up, which makes it the best way to find your correct dose and adjust as needed.

Hemp extract taken sublingually should be your first choice for daily migraine prevention.

Topical Creams

Topical hemp creams do amazing things for people with muscle and nerve pain, which is why they will help ease migraines too. Cannabinoid creams may even prevent migraines when applied to the face and neck areas.

The Trigeminal and Occipital Nerves

The nerve largely responsible for triggering migraines, the trigeminal nerve, is spread throughout the face. It's connected to the occipital nerve in the back of the head and neck, but can also be directly affected by shoulder and back tension.

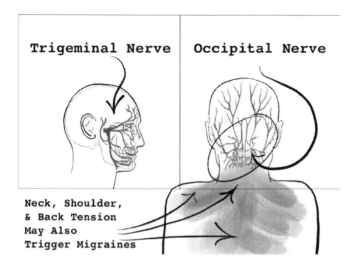

Alleviating pain in these nerves is the reason why Botox, nerve blocks, and electrical stimulation are successful at preventing migraines. Massage is also effective at reducing migraines, but some of that success may come from the secondary relaxation effects that massage brings to the entire body. Cannabis-infused oil massages are a thing in legalized states, such as Colorado, in case you were wondering.

Does THC Cream Get You High?

You might be thinking that a cannabis massage, with THC, would be an outer body experience. And it might be, but it won't get you high.

According to Dr. Alan Shackelford, a physician in Denver, Colorado, "Topically applied marijuana extracts have been found to be extremely effective for the treatment of pain, and do not exert any psychoactivity whatsoever."[132] Many cannabis manufacturers, such as Mary Jane's Medicinals, claim that THC from creams do not make it into the bloodstream and none of their customers have tested positive for THC after the use of topicals only. There are no reports to suggest that the company is mistaken, but I couldn't find any clinical evidence to tell you with 100% certainty that you'll pass an FBI background check, if you're on the market to join a government entity.

Transdermal Patches

Transdermal patches are a different story. They can get you high. Transdermal patches are designed to deliver a consistent dose of THC to the blood-stream. Patches may benefit migraine sufferers during a migraine because they bypass the gut and can start working immediately. Some transdermal patches are designed to deliver THC over an extended period of time and can have a similar effect to micro-dosing THC, which will limit side effects. Some transdermal manufacturers claim they use absorption methods that convert THC before it's introduced to the blood, but if you don't want to risk any THC entering the blood, a topical cream is a better choice.

THC Skin Absorption

There is an absolute benefit to using a cannabinoid cream with THC because it's anti-inflammatory and can further relax the muscles. Just make sure you get cream that first includes CBD. While topical THC is effective, CBD's topical absorption is 10-times higher than THC.[133] THC is one of the most potent anti-inflammatories, so it doesn't necessarily mean that CBD's higher absorption rate makes it superior. However, CBD is proven to block CGRP and you don't want to miss out on that.

Calcitonin Gene-related Peptide (CGRP)

The trigeminal nerve releases calcitonin gene-related peptide (CGRP) during a migraine.[134] Scientists began working on drugs that block CGRP to prevent migraines shortly after finding that CGRP triggered migraines when injected into migraine patients.[135] Unfortunately, the CGRP antibody drugs will cost an arm and a leg (with an estimated cost of $8,000 to $20,000 per year) and their side effects are likely problematic, according to a study titled "Wiping Out CGRP: Potential Cardiovascular Risks."[136]

Endocannabinoids and CGRP

CGRP is a peptide that is found throughout the body and may help regulate all major systems, including respiratory, cardiovascular, intestinal, and immune.[137] By this statement, you could guess that CGRP must somehow have a connection to the endocannabinoid system, and it does. Depleted levels of endocannabinoids are found in chronic migraineurs with high levels of CGRP.[138] A 2016 study published in the *European Journal of Pain* found that topical CBD can reduce CGRP, inflammation, swelling, and pain in animals with arthritis. The authors noted that this might be superior to oral CBD because absorption is much higher.[139]

Endocannabinoids also reduce some of the side effects of increased levels of CGRP, such as elevated levels of nitric oxide, which trigger migraines.[140] Just look at studies of Viagra, which increase nitric oxide in certain areas of certain older gentlemen, and you will find insanely high rates of migraines as a side effect.[141]

Guess what triggers the release of CGRP? You guessed it. CGRP is released from the exposure to oxidative stress or inflammation.[142] Geeze bageeze, this endocannabinoid research just keeps getting more intriguing. The endocannabinoid system controls oxidative stress and CGRP. Migraine sufferers have more oxidative stress and CGRP. We better fuel up that endocannabinoid system to prevent oxidative stress, CGRP, and migraines.

From the Face to the Shoulders

You want to reduce oxidative stress in the entire body, but those nerves around the face, head, neck, and shoulders are extremely susceptible. For example, a massive 55.3 percent of temporomandibular joint dysfunction (aka TMD or jaw pain) patients also had migraines in a 2010 study conducted in Brazil. Jaw pain promotes oxidative stress, which is sensed by the trigeminal nerve and is exceedingly common in migraine sufferers.[143]

The odds of experiencing migraine are nearly five times higher in people with spinal cord injuries, based on data from over 61,000 patients.[144] I can't tell you how many migraine sufferers have told me, "The first migraine I got was after whiplash from a car accident," or "My migraines got really bad after a neck injury." You don't need a car crash to feel stress in the neck or jaw. Any stress on the body, emotional or physical, will naturally tense up your jaw and neck.

A Vicious Cycle

The relationship between migraine and trigeminal or occipital nerve pain is not a one-way road, but more of a loop. Neck pain is one of the most common symptoms of migraine. Neck pain may increase inflammation in the neck or facial nerves to trigger migraines, but migraines also increase inflammation in those same nerves.[145] It's a vicious cycle and part of the path of a migraine detonating.

Just because you don't feel the inflammation, doesn't mean it is not there. This phenomenon is seen in migraine sufferers who benefit from Botox, even if they don't have neck or facial pain. Below is an image of the 31 injection sites of Botox for migraine prevention.

Botox Injection Sites For Migraine
(31 Total)

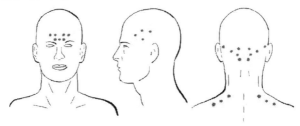

Notice how doctors inject Botox all the way down the shoulders, even though it's far away from the nerves associated with migraine, as well as migraine pain.

Botox temporarily paralyzes the muscles that compress the nerves, as well as other tissues that contribute to tension. As one migraine sufferer put it, "Botox is great for my migraines, but my kids think it's funny when I get mad because the top half of my face doesn't move." However, not all is well with paralyzing your temples. You know how the saying goes, "If you don't use it, you lose it."

One study found that out of 92 patients who underwent Botox for migraine prevention, all 92 experienced a deformity from muscle death in the temples.[146] Side effects such as muscle death may be why doctors do not typically inject Botox for migraine prevention into the muscles around the lower trigeminal nerve, which wraps around the jaw. You may want those muscles to work, for things like eating and communicating. Something that could relieve jaw inflammation without full paralysis or side effects may add to migraine prevention in a way that the Botox toxin can't.

Somehow, reducing the tension of the muscles around these migraine nerves can stop the cycle between migraines and facial and neck inflammation. This is why surgeons cut the muscle away from the trigeminal nerve and replace it with fat to decompress the tension and relieve migraines, a procedure called decompression surgery, which new research shows is absurdly effective for a small group of migraine sufferers who meet the criteria for this risky last-ditch effort.[147]

The Good News

The good news is that cannabinoids are proven to reduce oxidative stress, CGRP, overexcited nerves, inflammation, tension, and muscle pain. You can buy hemp and CBD creams or make your own by mixing CBD into your favorite facial cream. CBD is usually preferred in lotions because it is colorless and odorless. Hemp extract provides more cannabinoids than CBD isolate, but it leaves that earthy smell and yellow tint, which is weird, especially in public.

I can't write about cannabinoid creams without mentioning peppermint and lavender. Peppermint oil and lavender oil are the most popular essential oils added to migraine ointments.

Add Lavender

Several studies on animals and humans suggest that lavender has a calming effect that produces anti-seizure, anti-anxiety, and neuroprotective effects.[148] A 2012 study published in the journal

European Neurology found that lavender aromatherapy helped partially or completely relieve 92 out of 129 attacks in diagnosed migraine sufferers.[149] Another study published in the *Journal of Herbal Medicine*, in 2016, found that lavender therapy significantly improved migraine disability over a three-month clinical trial.[150] Adding lavender to your hemp cream may improve it, but peppermint is on a whole other level.

Add Peppermint

Peppermint's main ingredient is menthol, which is a key ingredient in most over-the-counter skin rubs used for pain relief and muscle relaxation. Menthol is a popular anti-inflammatory for the treatment of fibromyalgia and carpal tunnel, which are both linked to migraine. Peppermint oil is likely to slow the inflammatory response between the nerves in the face and neck, which cycle into a migraine. Make sure you avoid peppermint near the eyes, as it can sting and make you want to cry and say, *never again peppermint, never again.*

A 2015 study published by researchers at Thomas Jefferson University applied menthol gel on the neck and behind the ears of 25 patients during migraine attacks.[151] After two hours, 56 percent of migraine sufferers had significant relief and 28 percent had total relief. This confirmed a study by Iranian researchers, five years prior, which found that menthol was superior to the placebo in treating 118 migraine attacks for pain relief, nausea, sound sensitivity, and light sensitivity.[152] Peppermint therapy combined with hemp lotion will help CBD fight off migraines. Adding lavender to the mix won't hurt either.

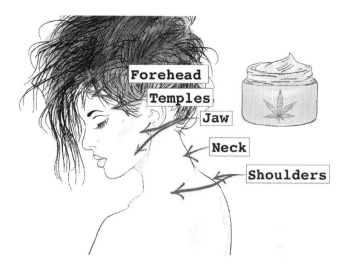

Cannabinoid Cream Summed Up

Use a hemp, CBD, or THC cream daily to relax the forehead, temples, jaw, neck, and shoulders or any other areas that you feel may be contributing to your overall inflammation levels. You can also use the lotion to reduce pain during a migraine by stopping the inflammatory migraine-nerve cycle. Applying CBD directly to the skin bypasses the stomach and quickly calms the nerves associated with triggering migraines.

HOW MUCH CBD DO I TAKE?

How much CBD do I take? The answer is displeasing: there is no one-size-fits-all dose. The endocannabinoid system represents your health, which is unique to you. The dose of cannabinoids that would benefit you the most is therefore specific to you and your health at any given moment. Luckily, there is someone who can help you find that dose.

Where to Turn?

Doctors won't have the perfect cannabinoid dosage when you walk in for your first visit, but they are masters of the dosage game and I always recommend you seek their advice for a cannabinoid dosage first. Doctors, however, will turn to someone who does know your perfect cannabinoid dosage, in time, and that someone is you.

This is the "take-two-of-these-and-call-me-in-the-morning system." The human body, your human body, is a state-of-the-art feedback system that is unmatched. When the endocannabinoid system is winning the battle against oxidative stress, the body rewards you with relief. The ideal hemp dose is the one that makes your body feel *consistently* great or at least *consistently* better.

Consistency is Important

The dose you take will ideally make you feel better immediately *and* that relief should continue without you feeling worse later. Consistency is important. Your endocannabinoid system is attempting to control your health by maintaining homeostasis, an equilibrium, a consistent balance.

The 2018 Washington State University study mentioned prior suggested that side effects, such as being ridiculously high, will not help with migraine prevention because "only treatments without disruptive side effects will restore normal activity."

Feeling worse off at any point after taking cannabinoids may suggest that oxidative stress is winning the battle against the endocannabinoid system. We want a cannabinoid dose that helps with long-term endocannabinoid function, for long-term migraine prevention.

The question is: how do you find the minimum dose that gives you the maximum migraine prevention with the least amount of side effects?

Start Off Slow

You don't want to start off with doses too high, because large doses of cannabinoids can have the opposite effect intended, increasing oxidative stress, inflammation, and possibly migraines.[153] [154] The body may also need time to adjust to cannabinoids.

Most manufacturers of full-spectrum hemp extract recommend starting off with low doses and working your way up until you feel terrific. For example, you could start off with 5 mg per day of CBD and increase your dose by 5 mg every week until you find your desired dose.

Starting off slow is the recommended way to go, but if 5 mg comes with absolutely no side effects, you want to try a higher dose on a day when you can afford to relax. Migraine sufferers are likely to need a higher dose than the average Joe and there is a good chance that you will feel better immediately. If you try a larger dose, such as 25 mg of hemp extract, and feel fantastic after, consider continuing with that dose or increasing 5 mg per week until you find your ideal dose. If a 25 mg dose comes with side effects or you don't feel your best self, reduce your dose.

Micro-Dosing

The risk of oxidative stress from high doses of CBD is relatively low. For example, there's not much harm in trying out 25 mg of CBD because the side effects are low and not likely to increase oxidative stress (100 mg doses of CBD or more are used in research, with no side effects). THC, however, is a different story.

For most people, 25 mg of *THC* is enough to get you high as a kite, throw off your equilibrium, and cause oxidative stress from the possible side effects. Hemp extracts are a safer option than cannabis extracts because they come with only one milligram of THC per 20 mg or 30 mg of CBD, depending on the brand. One milligram of THC is considered a micro-dose.

The general rule of micro-dosing THC is that you take as much as you can without feeling side effects, such as trouble thinking or drowsiness. Micro-dosing is usually under 2.5 mg of THC but can be as low as 1 mg for those who are sensitive to it, taken once or multiple times per day. I believe that hemp extracts come with enough THC for migraine prevention, but you may want to micro-dose additional THC if you have a high tolerance for THC or benefit from extra THC on a migraine day or when exposed to high levels of oxidative stress.

Migraine Attack

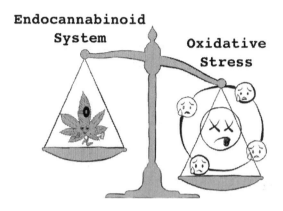

During a migraine, oxidative stress has outweighed the endocannabinoid system.

Migraine Prevention

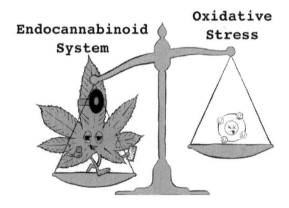

Migraine prevention happens when the endocannabinoid system outweighs oxidative stress.

The concern we have with THC is that its side effects may

contribute to oxidative stress levels. On a typical day, you may not want the side effects of extra THC, in addition to the amount of THC which your hemp already contains. For example, mental drowsiness could potentially create more stress, and oxidative stress, when you are attempting to perform mental tasks at work. Right? It's stressful when you can't think clearly at work.

However, a migraine day may justify the side effects of THC. A migraine attack comes with excessive amounts of oxidative stress to the body and central nervous system. THC relaxes the body, which is useful during a migraine attack. THC may be able to calm the inflammatory cycle during a migraine attack, which cycles between the central nervous system and tension in the face, neck, and body. It's cost versus benefit. If THC reduces more oxidative stress than its side effects bring, then it's worth it. Plus, the relaxation side effects during a migraine day may be welcomed if you are confined to a dark room and unable to work anyway.

In any case, you want to use the least amount of THC for maximum relief. Micro-dosing can help you get there.

The easiest way to micro-dose THC is with a cannabis extract that tells you the THC in each dose or drop. Remember that you want a cannabis extract that has CBD to counteract some of the side effects, or take a THC extract in addition to your hemp. Start off slow by taking a one-or-two-milligram dose of THC extract. Allow about an hour before considering an additional dose. As with CBD, there are too many variables and not enough research to give you a recommended one-size-fits-all dosage.

The way you micro-dose THC from an edible is not as scientific. You simply break the piece of brownie, cookie, or candy into smaller pieces. For example, you can cut a 10 mg brownie into four pieces to create four 2.5-milligram doses.

Edibles are food, and just like eating any food, can take up to three hours to fully digest, but may start to absorb in 30 minutes. Edibles are dangerous because you may think that you need another dose before the first dose kicks in.

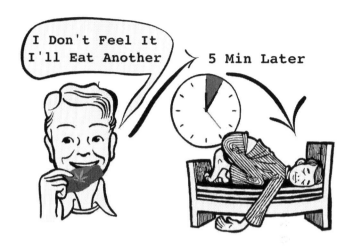

"I don't feel anything; I'll have another brownie." Five minutes later: "Uh oh, I feel the first brownie, I think I'll take a 3-day nap." Allow at least three hours after your first edible dose before considering another edible dose. Of course, this topic falls into the medical marijuana arena which is not the focus of this book.

Give Hemp Time

Some people will find that CBD will prevent migraines immediately or even abort a migraine that's already started. That's the best-case scenario, where you say, "omg, hemp has instantly changed my life. I love you, hemp. I need to go shout my experience from a rooftop." However, migraine prevention is based on reducing oxidative stress and it depends on how much of a reduction of oxidative stress you personally need to prevent the migraine threshold from overflowing. The endocannabinoid system improves your health, naturally, and that can take time.

In migraine research, most natural supplements or regimens are given a three-month trial to measure their usefulness, which is a reasonable amount of time to see if hemp will help you. Say that you work your way up to a cannabinoid dose that makes you feel good, or fantastic, or at least better; continue that dose for several months to see if it prevents migraines.

You can always up your dosage later or add other measures that boost your endocannabinoid system—which we'll get to soon.

What's Sondra's Dose?

Sondra, my wife, takes two 25 mg doses (one 25 mg dose in the morning and one 25 mg dose at night) of a full-spectrum hemp extract (Bluebird Classic 6x) to fight off anxiety and migraines. She can take up to 100 mg per day, on days where extra stress is a factor, without any side effects.

I only take 5 mg of the same hemp extract to feel great. Sondra is prone to migraines and likely needs more of an endocannabinoid boost than me. I would feel lethargic if I took 25 mg of hemp extract, yet she feels that it improves her total energy levels and mental clarity at her fast-paced tech job. My wife is tiny and I am large, in comparison. The dosage is not about size, but how much of a boost your individual endocannabinoid system needs at any given time.

Cannabinoid Doses in Research

Cannabinoid doses used in research are all over the place. Some studies show positive effects from CBD with just 5 mg of CBD, while successful anxiety and epilepsy studies range from 100 mg to 600 mg of CBD per day.[155]

If you just did the math on how much it will cost you to purchase and consume 100 mg of CBD per day, don't freak out. These studies are using pure CBD and aren't coming with the documented benefits of the entourage effect. You will not need as much CBD if it is coming from a hemp extract with multiple cannabinoids. Pure CBD is also much cheaper than a full-spectrum hemp extract if that's the route you go.

The recent migraine-cannabinoid study mentioned earlier, the one that outperformed amitriptyline in migraine prevention and also reduced the intensity of migraine attacks, used doses of 18 mg of CBD and 38 mg of THC per day. Amounts under 9 mg of CBD had no effect.

I suspect that using a hemp extract with high levels of CBD and low levels of THC would outperform this study. For example, Sondra's cannabinoid dose per day totals 50 mg of CBD, under 2 mg of THC, and a few milligrams of other cannabinoids. **I believe that 25 mg of hemp extract, twice per day will help many other migraine sufferers.**

Prevention Vs. Acute Migraine Relief

Based on the research in this book and testimonials from migraine sufferers, your optimal dosage of hemp extract for migraine prevention is likely to fall somewhere in between **15 mg and 100 mg of CBD per day**. However, a stressful day, a pummeled immune system or the consumption of headache triggers could immediately deplete endocannabinoids and increase your need for more cannabinoids. And a migraine day will indubitably require a higher dosage of cannabinoids for acute migraine relief.

The Cannabinoid Profile

It's not the size of the bottle, but the cannabinoid profile that is important. The cannabinoid profile is the quantity of each cannabinoid in a bottle or dose. A one-ounce bottle of hemp extract doesn't mean anything. For example, you could have 1500 mg of CBD in a one-ounce bottle or 100 mg of CBD in the same sized one-ounce bottle. You need to find out how many milligrams of each cannabinoid is in the bottle or dose.

The hemp extract my wife and I use has about a 30-to-one ratio of CBD to THC. That's 30 mg of CBD to one mg of THC. In addition, it also comes with small doses of other cannabinoids, which add to the entourage effect. The ratio is different for almost every company.

I believe that low amounts of THC and copious amounts of CBD and other cannabinoids is best. However, it is possible that you will benefit from a cannabinoid product with large amounts of pure CBD or THC.

What are Migraine Sufferers Saying?

This movement is growing fast and the testimonials are piling in. Go online to any migraine support group and ask if CBD has helped anyone relieve their migraines. Despite how many fake CBD products are on the market; you will hear from many migraine sufferers who have gained their lives back through the use of hemp extract.

The testimonials can also give you an idea of how people are using hemp and what brands/types to use. One migraine sufferer wrote to tell me that doses of 4 mg of hemp extract did nothing, but she experienced her first migraine-free month in years after using over 16 mg of hemp extract per day.

Another migraine sufferer shared with me her migraine diary, recorded in an app called Migraine Buddy, after using CBD for four months. My goodness, the results were fantastic.

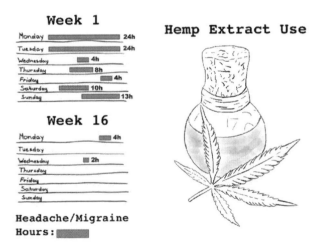

She started off with low doses and worked her way up to 50 mg per day, occasionally skipping days. The first week was typical for her, she had 87 hours of headache or migraine pain. By week 16, she had just six hours of headache or migraine pain, which was consistent with the rest of the month. I believe that if she used the other methods in this book to improve the endocannabinoid system, her migraines would go away completely. Her experience was incredible nonetheless and it inspired me.

A tipping point for me to research *Hemp for Migraine* was after I watched a YouTube review by Kelsey Darragh. Check it out on YouTube by searching: "I Tried Medical Marijuana for My Chronic Pain." Kelsey has a severe case of trigeminal neuralgia, which shares similarities to migraine. Medical marijuana didn't help Kelsey, but a hemp extract by the company Charlotte's Web did.

The combination of the research and hundreds of personal online testimonials lead me to believe that cannabinoids are something special. When you find out how hemp helps your headaches or migraines, share your experience on YouTube, or with a migraine support group, or with me at Jeremy@migrainekey.com. Sharing your personal experience is a powerful way to help people who are in a similar position, and it feels good too.

You've Got It

You now have the information you need to use hemp for migraine. This book will take a turn now to show you other ways to help hemp improve the endocannabinoid system, giving you the best chance of killing migraines once and for all. If you can strengthen your endocannabinoid system, you may not need to rely on hemp for daily migraine prevention.

Part IV: Fat, Hemp, and Brain Health

The following chapters reveal how healthy fats protect the brain from neurological disorders linked to migraine such as Alzheimer's disease, Parkinson's disease, and traumatic brain injuries. The research is more than impressive, and the migraine relief is unimaginable. As we move forward, hemp and endocannabinoids are connected every step of the way. This surprising connection could make your hemp unstoppable at migraine prevention.

AN INTRO TO FAT, ENDOCANNABINOIDS, & HEALTH

"The human brain is nearly 60 percent fat. We've learned in recent years that fatty acids are among the most crucial molecules that determine your brain's integrity and ability to perform," according to research published in 2009.[156]

New research suggests that you eat healthy fats, not become fat, for brain function, endocannabinoid function, migraine prevention, and health in general. Ironically, diets high in healthy fats such as the Mediterranean diet or ketogenic diet are associated with a reduction in excess body fat.

But before I put fat on a pedestal, we need to talk. It's about the fat myth.

The Fat Myth

A diet rich in healthy fats goes against what doctors, the media, our cereal boxes, and the food pyramid promoted for oh, about the last half-century. Every credible source told us that dietary fat would make us fat and unhealthy. Where did this bunk research come from?

According to a new study, not a news article or an opinion, published in the prestigious journal *JAMA*, the sugar industry created the disastrous fat myth in the 1960's after paying Harvard scientists to blame fat for heart disease.[157] It was a lie, and yes, it's always about money.

It wasn't until 2010 that the general public became aware that the old research wasn't adding up. That was the year that the *American Journal of Clinical Nutrition* published a massive review of over 300,000 people and 21 studies. The researchers found that there was no association between saturated fat and heart disease.[158]

Fat Myth Aftermath

We should have seen it coming. Let's look at the obesity rates from 1960 until now. The Sugar Research Industry sponsored its first study in 1965, in the *New England Journal of Medicine*, which slowly moved our eating habits away from healthy fats, and toward empty carbohydrates and processed foods. [159]

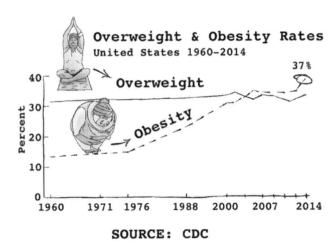

SOURCE: CDC

Do you see the problem? We told people to stop eating fat while we had a 13 percent obesity rate in 1960 and ended up with a 37 percent obesity rate in 2014.[160] I guess that didn't work. It's time we rethink the low-fat diet.

More than 70 percent of American adults are now, in 2018,

overweight or obese.[161] Remember that endocannabinoids maintain health and it becomes hard to do that when the majority of us are in the unhealthy category of "overweight." We need to save those endocannabinoids for fighting migraines, as opposed to fighting our own body fat.

What were we thinking? We should have looked over at the high-fat diet of the French in the 1990s and wondered why they had an obesity rate of just 8.6 percent, while the low-fat American diet was skyrocketing obesity rates toward the moon.[162]

We should have also wondered why France had a much lower migraine prevalence than the United States, with only about 8 percent of its general population suffering migraine versus about 14 percent of Americans. Only 11 percent of French women suffer migraine, versus about 20 percent of American women.[163] [164] [165] Maybe healthy fats have something to do with the low migraine prevalence and health in general of the French.

To be crystal clear, processed foods that contain highly processed fats such as vegetable oil or trans fats are not healthy for you. I immediately thought of greasy French fries the second I wrote this and thought, "How did the French stay skinny?" It turns out French fries are from Belgium. Healthy fats from natural sources are what the French were eating, and that's what your brain wants too.

The Fat Myth and Migraine

The fat myth and its push toward obesity have undoubtedly triggered many migraines.

Obesity is characterized by permanently increased oxidative stress levels.[166] Like clockwork, a recent study found that a dysfunctional endocannabinoid system may also promote the development of obesity.[167] You could guess what elevated oxidative stress levels and a screwed-up endocannabinoid system will do for migraines rates.

According to researchers at Johns Hopkins University, obesity increases the risk of migraines by up to 81 percent.[168]

A diet that includes healthy fats may lower the risk of obesity and thus migraine. But noticeably not all migraine sufferers are obese, of course, and the problem may start before or independently of weight gain.

Cardiovascular Disease and Cannabinoids

Obesity raises the risk of cardiovascular disease, which refers to conditions that narrow or block the blood vessels. Blocked pipes lead to heart attacks and stroke. I've seen a lot of those in the fire service. Cardiovascular disease is an ailment that takes more lives each year than any other illness or injury worldwide.

However, migraine sufferers have a 50 percent increased risk of cardiovascular disease, which is independent of obesity.[169] Yeah, that means skinny migraineurs also have an increased risk of heart attack and stroke. Why? Where does this increased cardiovascular risk come from?

Oxidative stress levels are a significant and well-studied factor in the development of cardiovascular disease. The common denominator here is oxidative stress, although the outcome of migraine, obesity, cardiovascular disease, and other chronic conditions vary. Oxidative stress is a predictable factor, but so is the rescue response of the almighty endocannabinoid system.

Recent studies have found that the cannabinoid receptor 2 has a protective role against cardiovascular disease.[170] A growing number of studies have found that CBD protects against stroke and heart attack in animal models and it's likely to protect humans too. According to researchers from the University of Nottingham, "a common theme throughout these studies is the anti-inflammatory and antioxidant effect of CBD."[171]

I know we should be happy that CBD fights the oxidative stress responsible for migraines and cardiovascular disease, but part of me is fuming that we waited so long to do the research. Most everyone knows someone who has had or does have cardiovascular disease, and we're just now looking into the life-saving research of this harmless plant that was demonized by jerks.

Even worse, we've had decades of observational and clinical trials showing that diets rich in healthy fats such as the Mediterranean diet protect against obesity, cardiovascular disease, and oxidative stress.[172] [173] However, the low-fat diet and its relics, such as "low-fat" stamps on processed foods, are still promoted by corporations and many nutritionists. Hopefully, the stigma against both healthy fats and cannabinoids changes, soon.

Fat, Oxidative Stress, and Diabetes

The focus here is not on how the fat myth promoted obesity and cardiovascular disease, but how a lack of healthy fats increase oxidative stress levels and hurt the endocannabinoid system.

Some people remain skinny when they eat inflammatory foods, but oxidative stress may still wreak havoc on the human body. For example, diabetes is characterized by increased oxidative stress levels and you can indeed become diabetic or prediabetic without obesity.[174]

Let's look at diabetes rates since the 1960s, when fat was deemed evil and we started eating more sugar and processed carbohydrates.

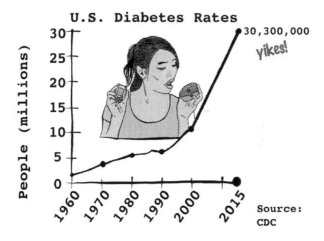

The above chart shows that there were a couple of million diabetics in 1960 and as of 2015 there were 30.3 million Americans with diabetes or as my paramedic partner called it, "sugarbeetes."[175] According to the CDC, another 84.1 million Americans have prediabetes.[176] That's over 114 million Americans with prediabetes or diabetes. There are only 250 million adults in the United States.

Great googly moogly.

Our American diet that is rich in processed foods and lacking in natural, healthy fats is killing us. What's it doing to our endocannabinoid systems?

Endocannabinoids and Diabetes

The cannabinoid receptors "influence glucose metabolism and are deeply involved in all aspects of the control of energy balance in mammals," according to a diabetes study conducted by Italian researchers in 2011.[177] (FYI, humans are mammals.) If endocannabinoids control metabolism, then the endocannabinoid system must be off its rocker when we have problems managing glucose, which is the case with diabetes.[178]

Diabetes is associated with an imbalance between endocannabinoids and oxidative stress.[179] New research suggests that poor endocannabinoid function may also lead to the development of diabetes.[180] Hold on, while I grab my bong to reverse diabetes. (Just kidding.)

Glucose is what your brain typically uses for energy during a process known as "metabolism." You can imagine that problems metabolizing glucose, our primary brain fuel, will not be suitable for brain health or migraine frequency. Migraine sufferers report hunger and low blood sugar as top migraine triggers, but migraines also have a direct connection to glucose problems.

Insulin is what your brain and body use to metabolize glucose into energy. Insulin resistance leads to diabetes and is associated with both obesity and chronic migraine. Surprise, surprise. However, a new study published in the journal *Cephalalgia* found that chronic migraine sufferers have higher levels of insulin resistance than non-migraine sufferers, even in those chronic migraine sufferers who are not obese.[181]

Insulin resistance may link to migraine because oxidative stress appears to be a factor leading to insulin resistance, even when obesity or diabetes is not involved.[182] It all comes back to the common denominator of oxidative stress.

Problems with glucose may become a problem for migraine sufferers, but this isn't about obesity or diabetes. It's about an equation: Poor endocannabinoid function + oxidative stress = migraine or conditions linked to migraine.

We want to find out how to solve this problem before it turns into any chronic condition, especially migraine. So, we are looking at how the low-fat diet contributed to poor endocannabinoid function and high oxidative stress levels for millions of Americans. More importantly, how can endocannabinoids and fat help the equation?

Numerous experimental studies have found that CBD is beneficial in the treatment of diabetes.[183] Go figure. Diets rich in healthy fats are also incredibly successful at treating diabetes, with one study finding that the majority of diabetic patients discontinued or reduced their medications after starting a high-fat ketogenic diet. [184] This research is wonderful. There are still many people who think that diabetes is genetic and there's nothing they can do about it. Healthy fats and cannabinoids beg to differ.

If healthy fats and endocannabinoids both attack diabetes, as well as cardiovascular disease and obesity, maybe we could combine them to attack the same problem that precipitates migraines.

Get Fat to Fight Migraine

We now know that healthy fats are needed for brain function and are likely to increase endocannabinoid function and reduce oxidative stress and migraines. The following research will not only prove it but show you exactly what happened to migraine sufferers who started a high-fat low-carbohydrate diet. The next couple pages contain some of the most inspiring migraine research that I have ever come across.

THE KETOGENIC DIET

The ketogenic diet is a high-fat and low-carbohydrate diet that allows your body to break down fat and metabolize ketones. Our brains run on either glucose or ketones. We just hashed over some of the glucose problems that obesity and diabetes cause, which lead to oxidative stress, endocannabinoid dysfunction, and migraines. What's up with this other brain fuel, ketones?

According to Dr. Peter Attia, a ketone expert, our bodies can't store more than about 24-hours' worth of glucose and we would all die of hypoglycemia if it weren't for ketones.[185] The body creates this marvelous fuel after fasting or when you are on a low-carbohydrate diet.

Ketones aren't something that we newly discovered from a fad diet. Think about how our ancestors lived. They didn't have 24-hour access to processed carbohydrates, and before agriculture, people would fast for days between hunts. The human body was in a constant state of ketosis (burning ketones for energy) from a low-carb diet or transitioned between ketosis and burning glucose, based on what carbohydrates were available seasonally.

Ketones are generated by a natural process in the body, but they can also be obtained by eating medium-chain triglycerides (MCTs) such as coconut oil, MCT oil, or grass-fed butter. Using ketones for energy is like turning off a sugar switch, which also gets rid of all the problems that glucose comes with. Before we explore the "why" of ketones, let's see what they do to migraines.

Ketones fight off migraines, forcefully. A case study published in the journal *Functional Neurology* in 2013 found that two twin sisters became migraine free after starting the ketogenic diet.[186] Yes, I did write "migraine free" and what's more impressive is that they were both chronic migraine sufferers before the diet, which means they each suffered 15-plus migraine days per month. Ouch. They tried the diet for three separate months in a one-year period and each time both sisters were migraine free within three days of starting the diet. Imagine their joy.

Check out their total migraine days for the entire year below. You can see that migraine days and migraine severity also went down during the months following each of the months that they were on the ketogenic diet.

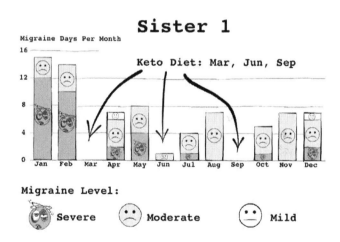

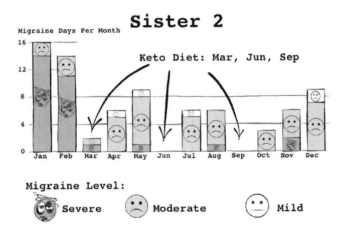

Migraine Days Per Month **Sister 2**

Keto Diet: Mar, Jun, Sep

Migraine Level:

Severe   Moderate   Mild

Note that the one or two migraine days each sister had in the months while they were on the ketogenic diet were at the very beginning of the month.

Ketosis takes about three days to kick in, so it makes sense that migraine relief also takes a bit of time. Improving oxidative stress levels and the endocannabinoid system can take multiple days or weeks, so you shouldn't expect such a quick recovery. However, I recently encouraged a chronic migraine sufferer to try the ketogenic diet along with hemp extract and she had the same speedy migraine remission as the sisters above. I was impressed. Not only at the miraculous results, but it takes a lot of willpower to start a strict diet with the promise of yet another "migraine cure."

Don't feel pressured into the ketogenic diet. We're going over the most successful migraine research that is linked to endocannabinoids to understand the relief process. We'll also look into how to use ketones without the ketogenic diet. However, we're not finished with the migraine success stories from the ketogenic diet yet.

A clinical trial of 100 migraine patients who took on the challenge of the ketogenic diet was published in 2013, in the *Journal of Headache and Pain*. The ketogenic diet incredibly reduced migraines in more than 90 percent of patients, which is far more successful than any migraine medication to date or in development.[187] Any given migraine-prevention drug will partially work for about half of those who try them—a coin flip—but most people need to try a few before they find one that works and deal with the side effects of each run.

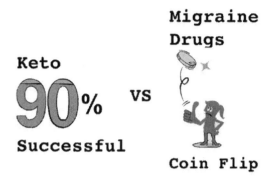

Keto **90%** Successful VS Migraine Drugs Coin Flip

It's one thing to have a migraine treatment that works well for a few patients, but it's something magical when it works for the far majority of migraine patients.

Similar results were replicated in 2015 and published in the *European Journal of Neurology*.[188] Ninety-six overweight female migraineurs went from a group average of 2.9 migraine attacks per month down to 0.71 attacks per month after starting the ketogenic diet. The most potent migraine prevention medications average about a 43 percent reduction in migraine frequency for an entire group.[189] [190] [191] [192] This study found a total migraine reduction of 75 percent, plus, patients reduced medication intake by 90 percent.

In other words, the ketogenic diet is way more successful than any migraine medication, ever. I can't imagine what the success rate would be if we combined the ketogenic diet with cannabinoids. Before you start the ketogenic diet, know that doctors and nutritionists helped patients in these studies. It's a difficult diet, one that I'm currently on. You should not make this drastic dietary change without learning more about the ketogenic diet and speaking with your doctor or nutritionist.

The Mitochondria

According to the lead author and arguably the most influential researcher of ketones for migraines, Dr. Di Lorenzo, the underlying mechanisms of the ketogenic diet responsible for migraine relief could be its ability to control neural inflammation and excitotoxicity, and enhance mitochondrial energy.

Let's get into some nerd stuff. I feel that if you made it this far in the book, we must be connecting on my nerd level. No? Well, you're still going to want to hear about this. The mitochondria create energy for the brain and fight off oxidative stress, so it makes sense that a brain fuel such as ketones would give the mitochondria power and prevent them from being weak. You don't want weak mitochondria. Migraine is linked to mitochondrial dysfunction, which creates oxidative stress. *Ain't nobody got time for that.*

It would be difficult to mention the mitochondria, the powerhouse of the cell, without mentioning the endocannabinoid system, which regulates energy. We know that migraine sufferers have low endocannabinoid levels and low mitochondrial function.

Guess where French researchers recently found the cannabinoid receptors responsible for regulating cellular energy? They found CB1 receptors on the external membrane of none other than the mitochondria, a finding that was published in the journal *Nature Neuroscience* in 2012.[193] That makes too much sense.

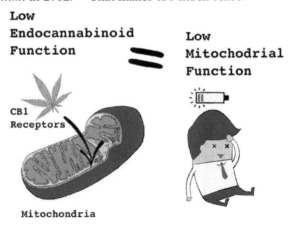

Low Endocannabinoid Function = Low Mitochodrial Function

CB1 Receptors

Mitochondria

The endocannabinoid system regulates the mitochondria. Migraine sufferers have low levels of endocannabinoids and therefore also have low levels of energy production by the mitochondria.

Mitochondrial Dysfunction and Fatigue

We're talking about cellular energy here, but it's the same "energy" as when you say, "I have low energy, I'm tired, fatigued." Fatigue goes hand in hand with migraines and is a symptom of the prodrome phase or "hangover" phase of a migraine. When fatigue never goes away, even with rest, it's called chronic fatigue syndrome.

Check this out; chronic fatigue syndrome is linked to mitochondrial dysfunction. The severity of chronic fatigue syndrome is also correlated with the degree of mitochondrial dysfunction.[194]

That's a simple concept: the worse off your mitochondria, the more tired you will be. And migraine sufferers are tired of being tired. However, this problem goes beyond fatigue.

Chronic fatigue syndrome can destroy your everyday life, but it is a double-edged sword when it comes to migraines. Two studies in the last decade have measured the relationship between patients with chronic fatigue syndrome and migraine. Both studies found that over 80 percent of patients with chronic fatigue syndrome also had a migraine diagnosis.[195] [196] That is an absurdly high percent of migraine sufferers, which I say as a person who reads migraine research all day every day.

The connection between endocannabinoids, mitochondria, fats, and energy production runs deep. Real deep.

Fun fact: Cancer cells feed on glucose and both research in animals and case studies in humans show that switching to ketones starves cancer cells, reduces tumor size, and improves survival rates.[197] Yes, this is a migraine book, but who wants cancer? Consider it.

CBD and Ketone Energy

The ketogenic diet, with its ability to increase mitochondrial energy, could help out in this situation. You would think that fasting or getting rid of carbs would make you feel tired. You might feel tired temporarily, but the increase in energy and mental clarity is surprising once your body is in ketosis and burning ketones instead of glucose.

I also believe this is why some migraine sufferers feel more energy after consuming CBD. If you have low endocannabinoid function, which controls the mitochondria, then it makes sense that you will have more energy once the endocannabinoid system is functioning at full speed.

One More Thing About the French

The French study which discovered that there are cannabinoid receptors on the mitochondria, known as mtCB(1), also found that those receptors are responsible for retrograde signaling. We briefly touched on this earlier. Retrograde signaling blocks glutamate. The buildup of glutamate is toxic for migraine and epilepsy sufferers, which is why medications that slow down glutamate are used to treat both migraine and seizures.

On top of placing glutamate in check, follow up research in 2016 from the University of Bordeaux, France, again, the French, found that the mitochondria cannabinoid receptors, mtCB(1), appear to regulate oxidative stress.[198] It always comes back to oxidative stress.

This is an important discovery because most of the research on oxidative stress is about identifying it and wondering where it came from or how we can get rid of it. These findings take us a step closer to figuring out how to battle migraines and a long list of chronic diseases.

What Did We Learn?

The ketogenic diet demolishes migraines in a high percentage of migraine sufferers. Ketones improve energy and increase mitochondrial function, and everyone wants more energy. The endocannabinoid system regulates the mitochondria and the cannabinoid receptors that live on the mitochondria block glutamate and oxidative stress. That's like a round-house kick to migraines, from Chuck Norris.

We may want to combine healthy fats and endocannabinoids, because they accomplish the same goal. The story gets even more exciting when we look deeper into how cannabinoids and ketones block glutamate, but we'll save that discussion for the next chapter on epilepsy and migraines.

Ok, a Final Thought on the French

It's ironic that the French made these breakthrough discoveries about the endocannabinoid system and the mitochondria, because France has some of the harshest anti-cannabis laws in Europe. One joint of ganja will cost you up to a 3,750 euro fine and up to one year in a stinky French prison. What? All prisons are stinky.

The French also have some of the highest rates of cannabis use among all European nations, with a recent survey by the French Observatory for Drugs and Addiction (France's government source of drug statistics) finding that 17 million French people have tried marijuana and 700,000 French people use it every single day.[199] Mind you that the French are contending with the cannabis use of other European nations like the Netherlands and Portugal, which have decriminalized pot, among other drugs.

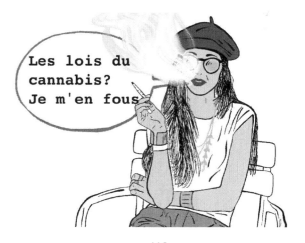

You would think that a year in jail would deter anyone from cannabis, but prohibition does not work. Cannabinoids have the potential to save lives, with the whole oxidative stress thing, and we should consider that while we evaluate nonsensical laws that serve no purpose and block something that could prevent many deadly conditions and the migraines that are associated with those deadly conditions.

But I digress. Let's get back to the positive healing capabilities of cannabinoids and ketones.

EPILEPSY, KETONES, & CANNABINOIDS

The ketogenic diet has successfully treated epilepsy since 500 BC and became popular in modern medicine nearly a century ago.[200] Ketones block the high concentrations of glutamate, think monosodium glutamate (MSG), that become a problem in both migraine and epilepsy and many other neurological conditions.[201] Glutamate explains a lot about migraines and how to avoid them with ketones and cannabinoids.

What's Glutamate?

Glutamate is widely accepted as the most important neurotransmitter for brain function. Reading this sentence, remembering it, and learning from it, is all made possible by glutamate.

Too Much Glutamate and Teslas

When too much glutamate is sent too fast from overactive nerves, it results in excitotoxicity or exciting brain cells to death. Excitotoxicity is like a five-lane freeway with bumper-to-bumper Teslas driving at 200 miles per hour and then suddenly the highway becomes a one-lane tunnel. The Teslas, being electric cars, crash spectacularly into the tunnel and create an electrical explosion called excitotoxicity.

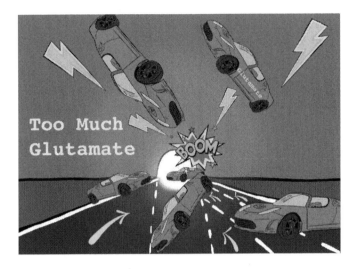

Some migraine and epilepsy sufferers can visualize excitotoxicity during an aura. The electric thunderstorm may start from just one synapse becoming blocked by glutamate. This electrical storm can be seen in CT scans as it moves from one side of the brain to the other. As this aura happens, sufferers may see a visual disturbance move across their field of vision. A migraine or seizure then takes hold of its victim shortly after.

Anti-Seizure Meds

Anti-seizure medication that blocks glutamate has been used to treat both migraine and epilepsy.[202] Ketones not only prevent this excess of glutamate but also reduce total levels of oxidative stress.[203] [204] Ketones do the same thing as the most potent medications, but without the nasty side effects.

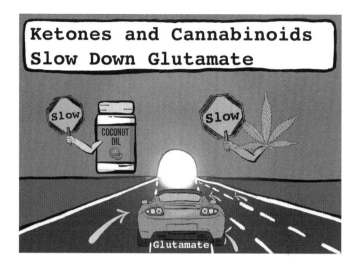

Do ketones sound familiar? As mentioned in the ketogenic diet chapter, the cannabinoid receptors on the mitochondria also prevent excitotoxicity and oxidative stress. Ketones do the same thing as cannabinoids, which is why cannabinoids also treat epilepsy. Let me introduce you to an influential little girl named Charlotte.

Charlotte

CBD is most famous for helping a girl named Charlotte who suffered from nearly 50 seizures per day. Charlotte's seizures were life threatening. After starting to take a hemp extract, Charlotte reduced her seizures to only two or three nocturnal seizures per month.

The University of Colorado published her case study and CNN later told Charlotte's story in a short documentary, which sparked a change in how we view CBD.[205] Charlotte is inspirational to millions, not just epilepsy sufferers and their loving parents, but to sufferers of any related condition.

Sixteen More Charlottes

Charlotte wasn't the first. A small study published a year prior, in

2013, by Stanford University, found that CBD-rich cannabis helped 16 out of 19 pediatric patients with treatment-resistant epilepsy. Forty-two percent of parents reported a greater than 80 percent reduction in their child's seizure activity, while 11 percent reported complete seizure freedom.[206] CBD is a life saver, literally.

One Hundred Twenty Miracles

Seizure relief is nothing short of a miracle, especially when all else has failed, a theme that continues in research. A recent study of 120 children with drug-resistant seizures found that CBD significantly reduced all types of seizures and cut the median frequency of seizures per month in half.[207]

Get Ready to Cry

Search on YouTube for videos of "CBD and seizure," and you will find CBD nasal sprays and hemp extracts immediately stopping active seizures in both children and dogs. It's astounding, but I warn you, you may shed a few tears after seeing a helpless child or doggy shaking uncontrollably before the CBD takes effect and calms the nerves. It's impressive how quickly CBD controls excitotoxicity, oxidative stress, and neural damage, which is why cannabinoids are also researched for Alzheimer's disease and Parkinson's disease.

ALZHEIMER'S, KETONES, & CANNABINOIDS

Alzheimer's is scary. At first glance, these seem like statistics that would make you want to put your head in a hole and avoid. But cannabinoids and ketones come in to save the day and they do it in fascinating ways. The links between migraine and Alzheimer's provide explanations and answers that will help avert both conditions.

Migraine and Alzheimer's Disease

Epilepsy doubles the risk of migraines,[208] but migraines may triple the risk of Alzheimer's disease, according to a study published in the *International Journal of Epidemiology* in 2001, which followed 694 Canadians over five years.[209] A follow-up study conducted a decade later by the Alzheimer's Association confirmed these harsh results.[210]

Migraines tripling the risk of Alzheimer's disease is inconceivable. We don't want to increase the risk of Alzheimer's by a single percent because the odds of developing Alzheimer's disease are not pleasant to begin with: one-in-three American seniors die with Alzheimer's or another form of dementia.

Women are particularly vulnerable to Alzheimer's disease, with a tripled risk of developing Alzheimer's over men.[211] You reading this book are more likely to be a woman, because women are also three times more likely to develop migraines over men.

The gender predisposition may stem from the mitochondria and likewise, the mitochondria may hold a solution to both conditions, even if you happen to be a man reading this book.

Mitochondrial Dysfunction

There is plenty of research that shows that mitochondrial dysfunction and oxidative stress play a role in the development of Alzheimer's disease for both men and women.[212]

Why does this problem, which is surrounded by the inability to metabolize energy, disproportionately affect women? In 2016, Singaporean researchers asked that very question. They wanted to know how the brains of women and men differ in response to Alzheimer's disease. The researchers found that women have more mitochondrial dysfunction in response to Alzheimer's disease than men, which they believed was responsible for the increased risk of Alzheimer's in women.[213]

The Singaporean researchers looked into the gender differences in how Alzheimer's destroys the mitochondria. But we are not looking for destruction. We want to know how to improve mitochondria function, especially in women.

Decades of research shows that men predominantly fuel the mitochondria with protein, while women predominately use fats as a fuel source within the mitochondria.[214] This basic research is staring at low-fat packages in every grocery store across America and saying, "Women use fat to fuel the mitochondria and fight off Alzheimer's disease, why are you trying to kill their mitochondria?" The war on fat may have disproportionately impaired the essential brain function of American women.

Maybe the mitochondrial dysfunction in Alzheimer's patients could give answers to the mitochondrial dysfunction in migraine sufferers, especially when it comes to women. Earlier, we looked at how diabetes and chronic migraine sufferers share mitochondrial dysfunction and how cannabinoids and ketones helped both conditions out. Alzheimer's disease might not be so different.

Type 3 Diabetes

Several extensive studies have found that type 2 diabetes patients are at risk of later developing Alzheimer's disease. Type 2 diabetes is when the entire body doesn't use insulin adequately and therefore has problems with glucose and energy. New research has found that animal models of both diabetes and Alzheimer's disease have nearly identical levels of insulin resistance in the brain. Alzheimer's produces a diabetes-like situation that is specific to the brain. The conditions are so similar that some researchers are calling Alzheimer's disease "type 3 diabetes."[215]

In Alzheimer's disease, there's a buildup of amyloid plaque in the brain. That amyloid plaque is toxic. Mitochondrial dysfunction is a hallmark sign of amyloid plaque buildup and may contribute to Alzheimer's disease.[216] The more amyloid plaque the brain has, the more the mitochondria struggle to absorb glucose, and the more damage occurs.[217]

The mitochondria absorb glucose with the help of insulin. They work together, so it shouldn't surprise us that conditions associated with insulin resistance such as Alzheimer's disease, diabetes, and chronic migraine, also have mitochondrial dysfunction. The links also establish a consistent need to nourish insulin and the mitochondria with healthy fats and a robust endocannabinoid system.

Type 3 Diabetes and the Migraine Brain

Alzheimer's disease is associated with white-matter brain lesions more than any other test or biomarker that could identify the disease.[218] Brain lesions are light or dark spots that show up on an MRI, which indicate damaged brain tissue.

Similar white-matter brain lesions are also more common in migraine sufferers than healthy individuals, although they share no direct link with the devastating memory loss of Alzheimer's disease.[219] [220] [221] [222] [223] An important distinction about white-matter brain lesions is that they occur before the presence of amyloid plaque and Alzheimer's disease.[224] We want to stop or reverse white-matter brain lesions at first sign before they cause any neurological damage.

Guess where white-matter brain lesions also show up? White-matter brain lesions indicate mitochondrial diseases or mitochondrial dysfunction.[225] If Alzheimer's and migraine share brain lesions, and mitochondrial dysfunction leads to brain lesions, and both conditions have mitochondrial dysfunction, then we should give the mitochondria everything they need to perform at maximum speed.

We also want the mitochondria to produce energy, so the brain doesn't shrink. If the brain doesn't have energy, you can't use it, and you may lose it. Yes, we are discussing the brain physically shrinking. But don't worry, we're going to use cannabinoids and ketones to prevent this bull hooey from happening.

Brain Shrinkage

Imagine that instead of giving a plant nutrients, you gave it poison. Instead of watering the plant, well, you didn't water the plant. The plant would shrivel up, and if you didn't do anything about it, the plant would soon die. That's what happens to the brain during Alzheimer's disease: the brain shrinks.[226]

Brain shrinkage isn't unique to Alzheimer's disease; it's what happens when there is mitochondrial dysfunction and the brain can't absorb nutrients, similar to the plant that you didn't water. There is brain shrinkage witnessed in patients with diabetes, obesity, and even in patients who have elevated glucose levels that are still in the "normal range."[227] [228] [229] Over 500 migraine sufferers were also found to have brain shrinkage when compared to thousands of non-migraine sufferers in a study published in the *Journal of Neurology* in 2013.[230]

Mind you that brain shrinkage from elevated glucose levels is happening to the majority of Americans who are on a low-fat and processed food diet. Brain shrinkage is common, but that doesn't mean it's normal. We don't want shrinkage, of any kind, so how do we avoid shrinkage and fatten up the brain?

Fat Fattens up the Brain

The brain is mostly fat, so consuming healthy fats from a Mediterranean diet would seem appropriate to keep the brain fat and happy. A study published in the *Journal of Neurology* in 2017 found that senior citizens who did *not* follow the Mediterranean diet had a more significant reduction in brain volume over a three-year period than those who *did* closely follow the Mediterranean diet.[231] There's also some preliminary research that showed that the ketogenic diet increased memory and brain volume in rats, although human trials are needed to confirm those findings.[232]

We don't need another study to confirm that fats fuel the brain and prevent shrinkage. We know through a vast amount of research that healthy fats and ketones avert neural damage, just like cannabinoids. We also know that glucose problems, diabetes, and obesity lead to brain shrinkage. If we remove the diets that cause brain shrinkage and consume nutrients that prevent brain shrinkage, we should be ok. Is that a sufficient answer?

"Should be ok" is not enough. Ketones, and also cannabinoids, need to prove that they can treat Alzheimer's disease if we are to believe that they can improve the mitochondria problems, brain lesions, and insulin issues that link to migraines. The proof is in the pudding. Let's see what happens when we add ketones to the pudding of Alzheimer's patients.

Keto Fights Alzheimer's Disease

Supplemented ketones and the ketogenic diet have been beneficial in both animal models of Alzheimer's disease and clinical trials with Alzheimer's patients.[233]

MCT oil, which is rich in ketones, has done something that drugs have failed to do for Alzheimer's patients. In 2004, published in the *Journal Neurobiology of Aging*, researchers found that MCT oil improved the memory recall of Alzheimer's patients.[234] Imagine that, we're spending billions on Alzheimer's research and something that comes from a coconut just beat every Alzheimer's drug ever developed. I can't believe that you thought less of all the people who use coconut oil as a remedy for every disease. Apparently, they were right about coconut oil and Alzheimer's disease before they had the hard science to back it up.

A patented MCT oil was also found to improve cognition in patients with mild to moderate Alzheimer's disease after 45 days of use, according to a 2014 study published in the *American Journal of Alzheimer's Disease and Other Dementias*.[235] Another win for MCT oil fighting off Alzheimer's symptoms. Hopefully, it doesn't take another decade for the next study to come in on this natural way to fight off Alzheimer's disease. MCT oil is attractive because it takes very little work to add to the diet, it's cheap, and it's available now.

If MCT oil is powerful enough to reverse the effects of Alzheimer's disease, imagine what it could do for migraine prevention. Alzheimer's researchers attribute the success of ketones in Alzheimer's disease treatment in the same way that migraine studies explain the success of ketones in migraine prevention. Both Alzheimer's and migraine researchers suggest that ketones work by increasing the brain's metabolism even in the face of oxidative stress or glucose problems.[236 237 238]

(I'll get to the nitty gritty results of MCT oil and ketone supplements for migraine sufferers soon.)

The results aren't in for the full force of the ketogenic diet on Alzheimer's disease. Studying Alzheimer's disease and the ketogenic diet is more complicated than studying the effects of just MCT oil because of all the variables involved. Plus, the ketogenic diet requires a significant change in lifestyle, which can be tough for seniors who like consistency. However, a recent study of 23 seniors with mild cognitive impairment found that their memory recall improved following six weeks on the ketogenic diet. Ketones were positively correlated with memory performance: the higher the ketone levels, the better the memory.[239] If you try the ketogenic diet, you'll be like, "Yeah, increased memory. I'm not surprised. My brain is firing faster than ever on the keto diet."

It's plausible that the ketogenic diet will be as successful at treating Alzheimer's disease as MCT oil has shown to be. The ketogenic diet raises ketones to higher levels for more extended periods of time than you could obtain from supplementation. It sounds like the ketogenic diet has the potential to be as successful in Alzheimer's disease treatment as it is for migraine and epilepsy.

A Fat Caveat

Starting the ketogenic diet after one develops Alzheimer's disease doesn't entirely measure its potential. Those studies disregard Alzheimer's prevention abilities. We need more research on the ketogenic diet and we needed it yesterday, or better yet, 24 years ago. I'll explain.

There's a reason that Alzheimer's is predominantly found in people over the age of 65; it typically takes years to develop. A new study by John Hopkins University School of Medicine followed up with seniors who had elevated levels of inflammation 24 years prior.[240] The researchers found that elevated levels of inflammation throughout the body at midlife resulted in higher levels of inflammation in the brain as well as losses of brain volume later in life. The areas of damage were signature to Alzheimer's disease.

We start planning for retirement young, at least that's the idea. We should approach Alzheimer's prevention the same way as retirement because money won't matter much if we are not conscious to enjoy it, plus Alzheimer's care costs American families more than a quarter of a trillion dollars per year. We need to battle the inflammation today that could snowball into Alzheimer's disease 20 some years from now. Migraines may be trying to tell us what research is now figuring out.

I previously described the headache threshold as a cup filled with oxidative stress and when it overflows, it triggers a migraine. Well, you might as well think of that cup of oxidative stress as a cup of inflammation, because with one comes the other.

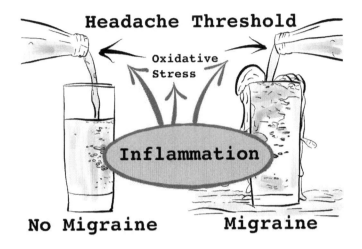

Headache Threshold

Oxidative
Stress

Inflammation

No Migraine   Migraine

Migraines triggered by inflammation today may be a defense mechanism against what that inflammation may turn into decades down the line. That's not to say that the inflammation will turn into Alzheimer's disease, but migraine may warn us of inflammation that may lead to a variety of potential problems.

Here's where endocannabinoids come back into the picture. Endocannabinoids regulate the immune system, which includes keeping inflammation in check. [241] If a stable endocannabinoid system can keep inflammation in check, or oxidative stress in check, or mitochondrial dysfunction in check, we may be able to stop the brain damage or brain shrinkage before it occurs.

Let's look at the breadcrumbs left by endocannabinoids in Alzheimer's disease research to find our way back to a healthy brain.

Endocannabinoids and Alzheimer's

One of the problems with studying endocannabinoid absorption in the brain is that you need to take a physical slice out of the brain to determine endocannabinoid levels. While there are probably some serious cannabis enthusiasts out there who have said, "Just do it, take a little slice out of my brain, in the name of cannabis science," studies of endocannabinoid absorption on live patients have yet to happen. However, there have been Alzheimer's patients and non-Alzheimer's patients who donated their brains to science after death to study endocannabinoid levels. The results are telling.

Researchers from the University of California found in 2012 that the post-mortem brains of Alzheimer's patients had significantly lower levels of endocannabinoids compared to the brains of non-Alzheimer's patients.[242] The areas with low endocannabinoid levels correlated with white-matter brain lesions and cognitive deficiencies. The results suggested that endocannabinoid dysfunction leads to cognitive dysfunction in Alzheimer's disease.

You are not surprised, are you? You know that with low mitochondrial function comes low endocannabinoid function. However, this confirms our need to improve endocannabinoid function in the migraine brain to avoid the shared white-matter brain lesions, and maybe migraines altogether.

The big question is, "Can cannabinoids prevent Alzheimer's disease?" CBD has been shown in multiple studies to not only prevent cognitive deficits in Alzheimer's mice models but reverse the effects of Alzheimer's disease.[243] A 2014 study published in the *Journal of Alzheimer's Disease* was the first to find that CBD prevents the loss of social recognition in Alzheimer's mice models.[244] If true in humans, that would be the difference between Grandpa saying "I'm so happy to see you," and "Who the dagnabbit are you?"

A 2015 study found that a combination of CBD and THC was able to preserve memory in early symptom stages of Alzheimer's mice and reduce the learning impairment witnessed in later stages of Alzheimer's disease.[245] The amyloid plaque associated with brain lesions was also significantly reduced and the researchers noted that CBD seemed to block all of THC's psychoactive effects.

Cannabinoids are reducing the problems in Alzheimer's disease, which correlate with migraines, in ways beyond what any medications have been able to do.

Alzheimer's Summary

By going over facts seldom discussed with migraine sufferers, because they are chilling, we discovered breathtaking migraine research. Sometimes the best way to find relief is to expose the pain, which you just read through like a migraine warrior.

Migraines increase the risk of Alzheimer's disease and both conditions may disproportionately affect women, possibly from their shared relation to mitochondrial dysfunction. Women fuel the mitochondria primarily with fats, instead of protein like men, which means the low-fat diet was an abominable idea for female migraine sufferers.

This chapter played out how insulin resistance, endocannabinoid dysfunction, mitochondrial dysfunction, oxidative stress, brain lesions, and brain shrinkage affect both migraine and Alzheimer's disease. Cannabinoids and ketones prevent all of these conditions, which may be why they treat or reverse migraines and Alzheimer's disease in new and exhilarating research.

PARKINSON'S, KETONES, & CANNABINOIDS

The following chapter is swift and to the point, much like the rapid effects of cannabinoids and ketones on the symptoms of Parkinson's disease. The Alzheimer's research covered in the last chapter established a formula for detouring migraines: reduce insulin resistance, mitochondrial dysfunction, oxidative stress, neurological damage, and brain shrinkage. All of these conditions are also linked to Parkinson's disease.

Enough said, you can assume from our simple formula that cannabinoids and ketones will benefit Parkinson's disease much like they benefit Alzheimer's and migraine. Since we already hashed out much of the science, we can dive straight into the shocking effect cannabinoids had on a guy named Larry.

Larry and Parkinson's

Larry is a retired police captain who sufferers from Parkinson's disease. He tried a marijuana-derived CBD oil for the first time and the results were spectacular. Words don't do it justice; you need to see it for yourself. Look up Larry's YouTube video called, "Medical Marijuana and Parkinson's Part 3 of 3."

Larry's Parkinson's symptoms are severe. Moving, speaking, and everyday life looks tough for Larry. In the video, Larry sits down and struggles to put the cannabis oil under his tongue. A few minutes pass by, and his symptoms appear to vanish. It's as if a switch turned off his overactive nerves and allowed Larry to do the things we all take for granted.

The Parkinson's treatments that Larry had tried in the past cost him hundreds of thousands of dollars, and they didn't work, but a CBD-rich cannabis oil did. The video gives you tingles and a feeling that there is hope in treating migraine with cannabinoids. But what is the direct relationship between Parkinson's and migraine?

Parkinson's Disease and Migraine

Migraine sufferers have a 64 percent increased risk of developing Parkinson's disease, according to a study of more than 41,000 people conducted by the National Taiwan University Hospital, in Taiwan.[246] Should you be worried? No.

Only about 0.2 percent of the United States population is estimated to have a Parkinson's diagnosis.[247] A migraine diagnosis would only kick that risk up to about 0.3 percent. However, the relationship between the two conditions is statistically significant and a quick look into Parkinson's disease offers a better understanding of how to prevent both conditions.

Parkinson's and Endocannabinoids

Parkinson's disease results in the death of the neurons that are responsible for controlling the motor system, with the most obvious symptoms of shaking, rigidity, and difficulty moving. That is Parkinson's in a nutshell and the endocannabinoid system has the opposite effect essentially, in a good way. The endocannabinoid system is neuroprotective and regulates the motor system.[248] We're fighting neurodegeneration of the motor system with neuroprotection.

Let's go one step deeper into the damaged nerves of Parkinson's disease. The overactive nerves found in Parkinson's patients have increased levels of glutamate, similar to migraine, which contributes to the excitotoxicity and oxidative stress responsible for their damaged neurons.[249] That's all we need to know, to know that cannabinoids and ketones will help. Cannabinoids and ketones calm the nerves and control excitotoxicity in migraine and related conditions such as epilepsy.

The deeper we go into the conditions related to migraine, the more fascinating it gets and the more we understand how cannabinoids can get to the root cause of migraines.

Cannabinoids and Parkinson's

There are a couple of recent studies that showed that CBD improved the symptoms of six or seven Parkinson's patients, just like it did for Larry. [250] [251] There's also a couple of small studies that showed that cannabis immediately benefited the motor symptoms of Parkinson's patients. [252] [253]

There's no other way to put this: the lack of clinical research on cannabinoids and Parkinson's disease is pathetic. Given what we know about the neuroprotective qualities of cannabinoids, we need large clinical trials now so that patients like Larry are given clinical proof of this life-altering treatment the minute they are diagnosed with Parkinson's disease.

Ketones and Parkinson's

A small study conducted in New York and published in the journal *Neurology* found that Parkinson's disease patients experienced a 43 percent reduction in symptoms after starting the ketogenic diet.[254] That could be the difference between dressing yourself in the morning or relying on a nurse to do it for you. Remember that the ketogenic diet helped control the overactive nerves in epileptic patients, as well as migraine patients, and now we find that it also controls the overactive nerves in Parkinson's patients.

Another study published in the journal *Neurology* followed over 5,000 Dutches for six years and found that those who consumed diets rich in healthy fats had a significantly lower risk of developing Parkinson's disease.[255]

All signs point to the benefits of consuming healthy fats before problems arise. Let's see what's happened to the rates of

Parkinson's disease as Americans started avoiding "evil" fats.

The Low-Fat Diet and Parkinson's

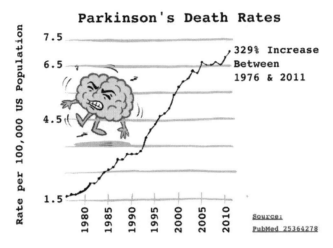

Parkinson's Death Rates

329% Increase
Between
1976 & 2011

Source:
PubMed 25364278

Above is a graph of Parkinson's death rates in the United States. There was a 328.7 percent increase in Parkinson's death rates between 1976 and 2011.[256] That's substantial considering this graph is based on death rates per 100,000 people and therefore accounts for population growth. Death rates are on the rise even though medicine has advanced.

The ominous incline of Parkinson's disease is on par with obesity, diabetes, and Alzheimer's rates after the introduction of the low-fat and processed food diet to the United States. The low-fat diet screwed all of the conditions related to migraine.

Sum it Up

Parkinson's disease has many similarities to migraine, including overactive nerves from excessive glutamate. We've seen the magic of cannabinoids abruptly calming the nerves in Parkinson's patients like Larry or epileptic patients such as the little girl named Charlotte. Ketones are surpassing the nerve calming effects of medications that are intended to treat Parkinson's, epilepsy, and migraine.

The more we learn, the more confidence we have that cannabinoids and ketones will combine to treat migraines. I've saved the most important ketone and cannabinoid results for last. The last condition related to migraine is up next and it's the most motivational for healing the migraine brain, especially if you played football.

TRAUMATIC BRAIN INJURY

We've peeked into the dark corners of conditions linked to migraine to find that ketones and cannabinoids protect the brain from harm. However, we can't appreciate this basic concept fully until we observe what blunt trauma does to migraine prevalence and what cannabinoids and ketones do to reverse this type of blow to the brain.

Migraines and TBIs

For a rat to sustain a traumatic brain injury (TBI) in a lab setting, researchers drop a 0.38-pound weight from just 30 cm above the rat's skull. That's all it takes.[257] It's sickening, but there is a much more violent experiment taking place across nearly every high school in America.

Children line up with their heads two or three feet away from the skulls of their adversaries and at the sound of "hut, hut, hike," they use the explosive power from muscles they've trained all season to plow through their competitors. Helmets clash with a thundering echo that ripples across the stadium. You remember your high school football games. After seeing some stars, the kids get up and do it again and again and again, and if they're lucky, they'll get a scholarship to hit their heads for higher education.

While multiple studies have found that TBIs increase the risk of migraines, some of the most influential of these studies are courtesy of football players. According to a study presented at the American Headache Society, fifty percent of high school football players who sustained multiple concussions also suffered migraines.[258] A concussion is the most common form of a TBI. These kids with TBIs had roughly five times the migraine prevalence of average kids.

Physical injury to the brain causes migraines, which narrows our approach to migraine prevention down to protecting essential brain function, hopefully with something stronger than a helmet. To take this experiment to the next level, let's see what happens to migraine prevalence when the biggest, fastest, and strongest athletes crack their heads against each other as a profession.

NFL Migraines

A retrospective study, published in the journal *Practical Neurology*, of retired NFL players showed that 92 percent of retirees experienced migraines. Wow, that's a bit more than 18 times the average rate of migraines in American men. That figure is almost as atrocious as the next statistic.

Thirty-six percent of players met the requirement for chronic migraine, compared to the 0.5 percent of men with chronic migraine in the general population.[259] Former NFL players had 72 times the risk of developing chronic migraines compared to the average American dude. Dude, I've read thousands of migraine statistics and this may be the most jaw-dropping.

Oxidative stress represents the damage that's triggering this insane migraine prevalence. Multiple oxidative stress markers increase and eight different antioxidant markers decrease after a patient sustains a TBI.[260] It always comes back to oxidative stress and we know what fights oxidative stress.

Get High and Don't Die

Cannabinoids may save your life, according to researchers from the UCLA Medical Center. [261] They investigated several years of TBIs at a level-1 trauma center, a top-notch hospital, and found that the mortality rate of people who DID NOT test positive for cannabis was 11.5 percent, while those who DID test positive for cannabis had only a 2.4 percent mortality rate. Great Scott!

To imagine this UCLA statistic another way, let's say a train carrying 1,000 non-cannabis users derailed and all passengers sustained TBIs. There would be 115 deaths. If all the passengers smoked a joint before the crash, there would only be 24 deaths.

Risk Of TBI Death

5 Times Higher When Not High

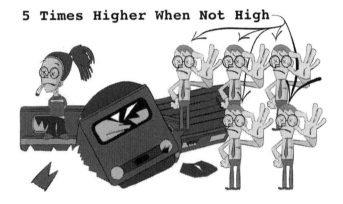

Your chance of dying from a TBI is nearly five times higher if you are not high, or at least do not test positive for cannabinoids. The California researchers attributed the neuroprotective effects of cannabinoids, which were demonstrated in several studies, to the higher rates of survival.

Note: This is an excellent time to reflect on the notion that cannabis is bad for your brain. In the above case, it prevented brain injuries, but the majority of people still believe that cannabis makes your brain... dumb. Joe Rogan: that's all I need to say. He often uses cannabis during his podcast—currently the top-downloaded podcast in the world—where he is a master at asking intelligent questions on a variety of complex issues. Rogan, like many, uses cannabinoids to enhance performance. Sure, some people get "stupid high," but others are using cannabinoids to outperform the rest of the human population.

Cannabinoids are protecting the brain from TBIs, oxidative stress, and death. Imagine their potential for migraine prevention. You know the drill, if cannabinoids help, so will ketones.

Ketones and Collisions

Research that was also conducted by UCLA Medical Center found that glucose absorption becomes weak after a traumatic brain injury and the brain may switch to its alternative fuel, ketones, for survival.[262] Multiple animal studies have found that ketones protect the brain after TBIs by reducing oxidative stress and increasing antioxidant markers.[263] That is exactly what we need to prevent migraines.

NFL and CTE

A recent study found that 99 percent of deceased NFL players had chronic traumatic encephalopathy, known as CTE.[264] CTE was also found in 21 percent of former high school football players and 91 percent of former college football players. CTE is devastating. You've probably heard of CTE from news stories about NFL players losing it or from the congressional study of the NFL suppressing the research, which was laid out in a biographical film called *Concussion*—watch it if you haven't.

CTE is caused by multiple TBIs and is behind the downfall of many players who become aggressive, confused, depressed, and suicidal. The signs of CTE are similar to other conditions that are associated with a substantial loss of brain cells, such as Alzheimer's and Parkinson's. The migraine links are all coming together now.

We're witnessing high rates of migraine in high school football players, which correlates with high rates of TBIs. As the years and hits go on, there's more brain damage and more migraines.

Retired Pro Football Players

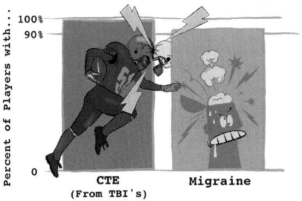

The incredibly high rate of migraines in NFL retirees—92 percent!—may be a defense mechanism that warns NFL players to stop hitting their heads before they develop CTE.

The outcome may differ (CTE, cardiovascular disease, Alzheimer's, etc.) but migraines are consistently there to warn us of oxidative stress before it may transform into a variety of deadly conditions. Of course, the oxidative stress is temporary and may not turn into anything. Migraines are measuring the temporary oxidative stress today to influence the healthy choices you will make tomorrow.

It's Not Normal

We all grew up with football and it's a socially acceptable sport. Some of us live for it. But repeated hits to the head is not normal. The rate of TBIs and migraine in football players is not normal. Right now, someone is throwing this book against a wall and condemning this research because of their unconditional love for football. It's ok.

We accept the things we become accustomed to, whether it's football, the low-fat diet, our anti-marijuana culture, or skyrocketing rates of conditions linked to migraine such as diabetes, heart disease, or Alzheimer's. It's hard to accept that we are wrong about the things we love or the conditions we have become numb to, but you are strong. You have looked into the scariest research possible for migraine sufferers and you are going to use this research to your benefit.

It's Time

We've looked into how conditions linked to migraine have increased with the low-fat diet. We've seen how those same conditions are reversed when cannabinoids and ketones are added to the mix. You've got the point. Now it's time you know why healthy fats are nearly identical to cannabinoids. Omega-3 is not going to blow your mind; it's going to heal it.

OMEGA-3

Hemp, you're so vain, you probably think this book is about you. In June of 2017, researchers from the University of Illinois made a breakthrough in the study of the human body: they found that the endocannabinoid system is not all about hemp. The team discovered that omega-3 fats also convert into endocannabinoids. [265]

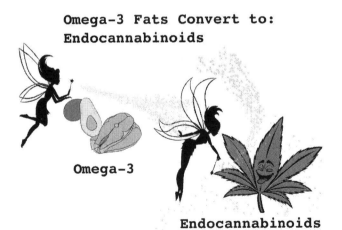

Omega-3 Fats Convert to: Endocannabinoids

Omega-3

Endocannabinoids

That's right, omega-3 fats create endocannabinoids, stimulate the immune system, and reduce inflammation as if they were cannabis, but without any side effects. Case closed. Your fight to destroy migraines with endocannabinoids just gained an entire army of healthy fats, but don't throw away your hemp just yet.

Omega-3 in Context

You previously read that omega-3 fats increase the absorption of the cannabinoids that you ingest by up to three times. Great success. Now, we learned that omega-3 goes a step further and creates endocannabinoids all by its lonesome self. This whole book has been about how endocannabinoids are supercalifragilisticexpialidocious at preventing migraines and so are omega-3 fats because they are one-in-the-same.

There's more. I'm about to hit you with some mind-boggling research: Omega-3 fats activate ketones.[266]

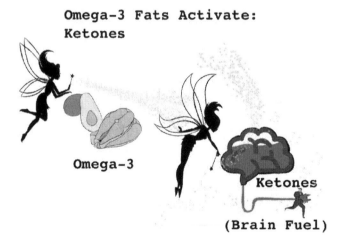

Omega-3 Fats Activate:
Ketones

Omega-3

Ketones

(Brain Fuel)

The last few chapters have been about how ketones fight migraines in a similar fashion to how endocannabinoids fight migraines. Migraines should be scared of omega-3 fat because it will attack migraines with both ketones and endocannabinoids. The question is, "How well do omega-3 fats attack migraines?"

Omega-3 Migraine Research

Several studies have found that increased consumption of omega-3 fats resulted in fewer migraines. [267] [268] A recent study by the National Institute of Health (NIH) increased the omega-3 intake and decreased the omega-6 intake of 56 chronic headache sufferers, 93 percent of whom had a migraine diagnosis. [269]

Average headache hours per day steadily dropped from 10 hours to less than four hours per day by the end of the three-month study. The decline in migraine frequency up until the last day of the three-month study suggests that these previously chronic migraine sufferers (having 15 plus migraine days per month) would continue to gain their lives back if they kept up their consumption of healthy fats.

Maybe you were expecting omega-3 to come after migraines like the Terminator, with all the force of ketones and endocannabinoids. However, it's more like a little ankle-biter dog relentlessly tiptoeing migraines out of your house. There's more to migraine prevention than just omega-3, but we should give omega-3 the credit it deserves.

Omega-3 drastically improved the lives of chronic migraine sufferers while they were on medications that commonly trigger chronic migraines, an event known as medication overuse headaches (MOH). It's likely that omega-3 would have slain more migraines if the medications weren't holding it back. This study also didn't remove any of the major migraine food triggers. All in all, omega-3 did phenomenal as a single resource for giving chronic migraine sufferers a significant portion of their lives back.

The Best Omega-3 Diet

May I introduce the ketogenic diet as the most successful omega-3 diet for migraine. You haven't forgotten about the twin sisters who became migraine free after the ketogenic diet or the study of 100 migraine patients, which had over 90 percent of patients drastically reduce their migraine frequency while on the ketogenic diet.

On the ketogenic diet, 70 to 90 percent of daily calories are consumed from fat. The ketogenic diet is abundant in omega-3 fats and low in processed foods with omega-6 fats. The first day you start the ketogenic diet, you'll notice that it's necessary to avoid most of everything in a package, because of all the hidden carbohydrates and sugar, thus, you'll naturally avoid most highly processed omega-6 fats.

The ketogenic diet removes most of the processed foods that trigger migraines, while we absorb omega-3 fats, ketones, and endocannabinoids. Hemp, this book is still about you, omega-3 too, and you as well, ketones, and anything that increases endocannabinoids or decreases oxidative stress. Migraine health is a combined effort. With that said, there are a couple more unique advantages you can get from omega-3 fats.

Omega-3 and Oxidative Stress

Omega-3 activates a switch in the brain called Nrf2, which might as well be called the antioxidant switch. Researchers physically deleted this switch from mice to see what would happen if they sustained a TBI. After the injury, the mice without this antioxidant switch had more brain damage and higher oxidative stress levels compared to healthy mice. [270]

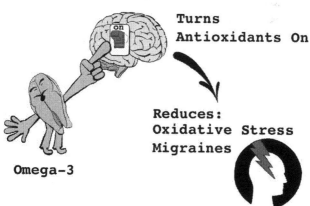

A 2017 study published in the journal *PLOS ONE* confirmed that omega-3 fats also reduce oxidative stress in human cells by turning on the Nrf2 switch.[271]

Oxidative stress is the master switch for turning migraines on. Put some tape on that switch that says "don't touch!" This antioxidant switch, Nrf2, which is flipped at the hand of omega-3 fats, must, therefore, be a switch that turns migraines off. Oh, and it is.

Research published in *The Journal of Headache and Pain* in 2016 found that indeed the Nrf2 switch completely prevented the trigeminal nerve from becoming overexcited, which triggers migraines.[272] I know that these researchers say, "We need more research to confirm these findings, so please fund the rest of my PhD." We already know what the Nrf2 switch will do to migraines.

Oxidative stress is the universal migraine trigger and omega-3 fats turn off that universal migraine trigger. We know this, but we should still fund that PhD's research so that the rest of the world's migraine sufferers become aware of omega-3. Or as kids would say, become "woke." I think.

Omega-3 Vs. Omega-6

Both omega-3 and omega-6 fats are essential fats necessary to absorb fat-soluble vitamins which fight off migraines, such as vitamin D. Endocannabinoids are also synthesized from both of these two essential fatty acids.[273] So why are we, and migraine researchers, avoiding omega-6 fat?

Grotesque amounts of omega-6 fat from processed foods are linked to inflammation, obesity, heart disease, and now, migraines. Too much of a good thing, omega-6 fat, can be a bad thing. Humans evolved with about a one-to-one ratio of omega-6 to omega-3 fat. However, most Americans, on our processed-food diets, eat about 25 times more omega-6 fat than omega-3 fat.[274] It's no bueno.

Pro tip: Find out how the average Americans live their lives today and don't live like that. Live like your grandparents did but pretend they approved of cannabis.

Don't worry about natural foods with healthy amounts of omega-6 fat. Just limit the processed foods that contain outrageous amounts of omega-6 fat, such as corn oil, vegetable oil, and most packaged foods. The same goes for other fats. Highly-processed fats become oxidized and lose their antioxidant ability.

Eat Natural Omega-3 Foods

Eating organic foods will help increase your omega-3 intake. Grass-fed and organic meats contain two to five times more omega-3 fat than grain-fed meats.[275] Some of the foods rich in omega-3 fat are flaxseed, salmon, chia seeds, walnuts, mackerel, beef, spinach, sardines, cauliflower, basil, broccoli, and arugula. Fish oil or krill oil are ultra-high in omega-3 fat, but make sure your supplement is high quality.

Sum it Up

Omega-3 fat is a switch that turns on ketones, endocannabinoids, and antioxidants. You could also think of omega-3 fat as a giant master switch that turns off migraines. To be fair, the migraine research suggests it is more like a dimmer switch that slowly turns migraines off. However, you could help omega-3 fats turn that migraine switch all the way off by increasing other sources of ketones, endocannabinoids, and antioxidants.

Bonus Tip

A 2006 study published by the University of Pittsburg found that 59 percent of patients with neck and back pain stopped taking their prescription pain medication in favor of an omega-3 supplement, fish oil, after 75 days of consumption.[276] They stopped taking their prescription meds because omega-3 pain relief was that good. Neck pain and back pain are top migraine triggers, and prescription-level pain relief is a bonus.

Omega-3 fat might not cure your migraines overnight, but give it time and it will move you toward migraine freedom, at a turtle's pace. Just remember a sea turtle moves like… a turtle, until it makes it to the water. Once sea turtles are in their ideal environment, they can swim at up to 22 mph. Omega-3 fats might get you to your perfect environment slowly, but you'll feel dashing once you get there.

If it's a speedy recovery you're looking for, look no further than the next chapter.

KETONE SUPPLEMENTS

When you start the ketogenic diet, your body produces ketones in about three days from natural sources of fat. Fasting is a similar process that accelerates the production of ketones from your own body fat. Both of these methods for kicking off ketosis can be a rough ride, but there's another option.

You didn't buy this book to paddle upstream. You are using hemp as an easy way to fight migraines by energizing the endocannabinoid system, which would otherwise be difficult to accomplish. Ketone supplements are like your second crutch, hemp under one arm and ketones under the other, that will help steer your endocannabinoid system toward migraine relief.

You can supplement ketones on their own or use them to make life a whole lot easier while stepping into ketosis.

MCTs

Eating MCT-rich foods such as grass-fed butter, coconut oil, and MCT oil may reduce migraines in the same way as the ketogenic diet, to a lesser degree. Unlike most natural fats or longer-chain fatty acids, medium chain triglycerides (MCTs) skip a step of absorption and are quickly converted by the liver into ketones.

MCTs are found to improve brain health, reduce oxidative

stress, and one study even found that adding less than an ounce of MCT oil per day to patients' diets resulted in improved weight loss.[277] [278] The combined MCT oil research suggests that MCTs will fight migraines by raising ketone levels, not as much as being in a constant state of ketosis, but enough to make a difference.

Ketones in a Glass

The goal of the ketogenic diet, fasting, or consuming MCTs is to increase the ketones in the blood, which boosts the endocannabinoid system's fight against migraines. The ketones in the blood are measured by beta-hydroxybutyrate (BHB) levels, and I just pricked my finger to see what my levels are.

My ketone meter, a Precision Xtra, shows 3.2 mmol/L. I'm deep into ketosis and I feel euphoric and mentally clear. I've been back on the ketogenic diet for three weeks now, but my ketone levels are higher than usual because I cheated. I just drank a glass of BHB.

BHB supplements have been in development for a long time and they're finally on the market. The one I just gulped down is called "Keto Drive BHB Salts," which I bought on Amazon because I'm an Amazon junkie.

For reference, light ketosis starts at a BHB level of 0.5 mmol/L, and 1.5 to 3.0 mmol/L is optimal for weight loss and mental clarity. Measurement can vary per individual and some people who are deep into ketosis won't have many ketones in their blood because their cells are efficient at absorbing ketones, but those particulars are for another day.

BHB supplements are expensive, but boy do they work. In the photos on the next page, you can see that at 11:03 a.m. I had a ketone level of 1.8 mmol/L. At 11:06 a.m., I slammed a glass of Keto Drive. One hour later, my ketones skyrocketed to 3.2 mmol/L. There are a few other brands you can try, but this one had great reviews on Amazon for the taste.

Ketone Blood Levels

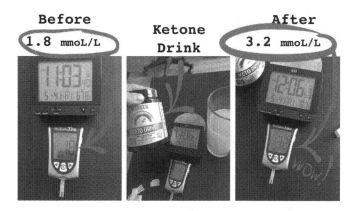

Before
Ketone Drink
After

1.8 mmoL/L
3.2 mmoL/L

BHB is a complete bio hack that bypasses all of the ketone absorption and conversion that the body naturally goes through and dumps pure ketones straight into the blood. Are you wondering what BHB supplements could do for migraine sufferers who are still enjoying all the carbohydrates that their hearts desire? Of course, you are.

BHB and Migraine Research

I'm excited to tell you that a new study presented at the 18th Congress of the International Headache Society 2017 looked into what BHB ketones could do for migraine sufferers.[279] Researchers gave four migraine sufferers 10 grams of a BHB ketone supplement (I just drank a 14-gram scoop and feel stellar) twice per day for one month. Something changed.

Average migraine frequency for the group dropped from 16 days per month to eight days per month. These are super impressive results in just one month because as the lead author notes, migraine days are likely to continue to drop for 90 days or more.

Four migraine sufferers aren't sufficient, but by the time you read this, the second part of this study may be published. Currently underway, researchers are giving ketone supplements to 90 migraine patients, twice per day for three months. I expect the results of ketone supplements to be better than any migraine drug ever produced.

I Do it All

I routinely will hop on the ketogenic diet and use a ton of healthy fats and MCTs to get there without having an emotional breakdown from carbohydrate withdrawal. I'd like to say I'm joking about the emotional part, but I get irritable while starting keto without the help of ketone supplements. Hemp also helps this whole process.

Should you do it all? That is a question for you. Do what you feel like and can get away with to feel great. Maybe you can get away with only using a little hemp now and again to boost the endocannabinoid system or maybe you want to go nuts and do everything and feel all amped up like I am right now. Of course, just because it works for me doesn't mean it's for you and always run changes this big by your doctor or nutritionist.

A FAT CONCLUSION

You just learned how ketones and healthy fats assist the endocannabinoid system in fighting migraines and conditions associated with migraines. Healthy fats not only triple cannabinoid absorption but are building blocks of endocannabinoids.

We learned how this combination of cannabinoids and ketones protect the basic health of the brain from the destruction that lingers around migraine. This fat-hemp duo shows more promise as a migraine treatment than anything on earth, in my humblistic—not a real word—opinion.

The choice of adding in healthy fats to your hemp regime or going full boar ketosis is up to you. But if you choose ketosis, you need to learn a bit more about it. Yeah, you could just eat less than 20 grams of carbs per day and you'll be in ketosis in several days. However, there are tips and delicious recipes that can make the process easy and fun, yes fun, I'm having fun feeling good and eating well.

(Oh, yeah, and talk to your doctor first because of X, Y, and Z, and don't sue me. ;))

Ruled.me or a dozen other free websites have fantastic guides that give you everything you need to know about the ketogenic diet.

There are also apps such as "Carb Manager" that will take all the thinking out of how to count carbohydrates and stay in ketosis.

Sondra, my wife, and I are currently on the ketogenic diet without eating dairy, with the exception of grass-fed butter and Ghee. This restriction narrows down our recipe selection. You'll find boatloads of keto recipes online are loaded with cheese and they are delicious too if you can handle them.

Some 75 percent of the world has some form of lactose intolerance and we both fall into that category. It's also a top migraine trigger. However, migraine health is individualized and just because Sondra can't have too much dairy, or she will get a migraine, doesn't mean that you will. It's all based on the headache threshold and many people do just fine on the ketogenic diet, from research and testimonials, even though most people eat dairy and other top migraine triggers like cured bacon while on the ketogenic diet.

Update: the allergenic problems that Sondra had with dairy and the gut issues that I had from dairy went away while we were on the ketogenic diet. We're both amazed by the results.

Diet is so successful at treating migraines because of the headache threshold. It's a big part of migraine health. If you are already eating a lot of natural foods and using hemp, you may not want to or need to go on any restrictive diet. However, if you want to do everything possible to stop migraines through nutrition, or at least be aware of the common migraine triggers and preventive foods, I've got you covered in the next chapter.

BONUS DIET

We're boosting the endocannabinoid system to beat down the oxidative stress that triggers migraines. At least, that's the goal. Some of the most common migraine triggers can raise oxidative stress levels beyond what hemp is capable of handling. For example, if Sondra—you remember, my wonderful wife—has too much dairy over too many days, it will predictably trigger migraines.

She didn't know that dairy was her migraine culprit for years because the most common food triggers are called IgG allergens. They average two-to-three days to trigger migraines and they can combine with other migraine triggers to do so. "Was it the wine or cheese that triggered my migraine?" It could have been both. Food triggers are part of the headache threshold and they can add up over a period of days.

Earlier in this book I talked about diets which resulted in complete migraine remission in up to 89 percent of patients. Imagine if we combined cannabinoids, ketones, and a diet that removed oxidative stress and boosted antioxidants. That combo would be the best migraine therapy ever, but it would require a lot of discipline and effort, and we're not all angels. You are the one to decide how far you want to take your migraine prevention efforts and then see what you can get away with once you are migraine free.

The first book I wrote about migraines was 500 pages and

focused primarily on migraine nutrition. There's a lot to learn about diet and migraine. After about five years, I refined the majority of migraine-diet studies into a single-page food overview and a 92-page PDF with all of the research cited. If you didn't notice, I like to be thorough.

What continues to astonish me is that there are over 1,000 cited studies, mostly PubMed, in my first book, PDF, and now hundreds more in this new book that your eyes are currently feasting on, and all the research is consistent with one theme: reduce oxidative stress to reduce migraines.

If you think I'm about to give you all my years of hard work for free, you're right. However, this is not the time nor the place. You can download the summary of all my work, *The 3-Day Migraine Diet*, for free, at migrainekey.com.

For those of you thinking, "I care not about diet, but maybe I'll try some of it out if you tell me what to do in a couple of sentences, maybe, but then get back to my hemp because you are stressing me out by trying to take away my pizza and cheesy bread, and the ranch I like to dip it into when no one is looking." Ok, pull my arm. I'll give you the quick gist of the most powerful migraine diets in research, and then we'll get back to cannabinoids because there are still other brilliant ways that cannabinoids fight off migraines.

I'll break the diet into three steps.

Step #1. Reduce the Top Food Triggers

This is the most crucial step in all of the studies that completely eliminated migraines in the overwhelming majority of patients.

The top migraine triggers, drum roll please, are: **milk products, wheat products, sugar, artificial sweeteners, and processed foods**. You do this step—reduce or eliminate the food groups above—and the research proves that you will have a great shot at migraine freedom. It's oversimplified, but it strategically covers the most potent migraine triggers. You'll need to read *The 3-Day Migraine Diet* to understand why.

Artificial sweeteners and milk products are very common migraine triggers that people use while on the ketogenic diet. I would avoid them while in ketosis, however, the ketogenic diet may be powerful enough, especially with cannabinoids added, for you to get away with consuming these triggers. Remember that you're working with a headache threshold and you can experiment to find out what actions will improve your specific headache threshold for eliminating migraines.

Step #2. Record Foods in a Migraine Diary

A needle in a haystack: that's what you are searching to find. When someone has a medical emergency, the needle in the haystack is also what the first responders attempt to find. We'll ask questions like, "What have you had to eat or drink today, or yesterday. What were you doing before you felt this way? Has this happened before?" And so on.

We are trying to find a pattern that triggers a medical event, in this case, migraines. However, finding migraine triggers can be nearly impossible if you don't write down the foods and events that led up to a migraine.

The haystack is humongous and we're actually looking for multiple needles. Because the most common food triggers are IgG allergens, we need to look at the foods and events that took place two-to-three days before you experience a headache, migraine, gut problems, or any time that you don't feel great.

The needles we're looking for don't always prick the skin. Some days you may be able to have wine. Some days you may be able to have cheese. Some days you may even be able to have wine and cheese. However, you might find that every time you have a stressful week and end it with some wine and cheese on a Friday night all hell breaks loose with a Saturday-morning migraine.

That was just an example, but you may have individual food triggers that provoke IgG allergic responses from virtually any food and/or only when combined with other triggers.

What did you have for breakfast three days ago and how did you feel that day? Exactly. It's hard to find the needle in the haystack if you don't remember what the haystack looks like. Even if you have the memory of an elephant, the most difficult problems to solve in life become a lot easier when we write them down and can see the entire equation. Over time you will see the same equation equal a migraine, over and over. The pattern will emerge.

Once you find the trigger, you remove it from your life and never look back. You hear me? Never! I'm just kidding. While it's logical to remove a source of pain, the headache threshold and migraine diary are about the ability to identify the problem and respond on your terms.

Say that you're a college student and get a migraine after the days that you are public speaking, which makes you a bit nervous but not enough to admit to anyone, and your migraine diary shows that you also happen to eat some comfort food leading up to that slightly nervous feeling: your migraine diary will not tell you to quit school and stop eating comfort foods. You are going to decide how to deal with the stress and foods that are migraine triggers. Or maybe you can take a little extra hemp before this whole debacle happens and perhaps that's all it will take to reduce your migraines. Once you identify the problem, you can decide how to solve the problem.

A migraine diary, which can be as simple as writing your daily events, feelings, and foods in a journal, can be of immense help in the creation of a personal migraine elimination strategy that's unstoppable.

Step #3. Eat an Abundance of Natural Foods

Oh, this step sounds easy until you walk into a grocery store and realize that 90 percent of the food is processed. That's one perspective. Another perspective is to think about explaining this struggle, and the struggle is real, to people in parts of the developing world who farm for survival, where the threat of modern-day starvation becomes real when crops routinely become scarce, due to factors outside of their control.

Yet, I think about how hard my life is when I walk through my grocery store in the middle of winter, surrounded by aisles of beautiful and disease-free meats, vegetables, and incredible seasonings. And that's about the time when I freak out because I have realized that there are only two cashiers in the whole store, who are taking their sweet time. Unbelievable.

Eating well is a struggle, but that's because we're spoiled to a point that would be inconceivable to our ancestors and, unfortunately, even to some people living today.

I promised you a quick summary, so here it is: eat foods that promote antioxidant levels in the blood. These antioxidant foods will attack oxidative stress, leaving your endocannabinoids available for attacking migraines. To fully appreciate the following list, you'll need to read the diet and learn about all the processed foods which raise oxidative stress, even though they proclaim "antioxidants" on their packages. It's not just blueberry muffins; there are plenty of foods marketed as "healthy," which only turn into oxidative stress in your body.

Here is a quick overview of the foods you should eat:
- Eat fresh, organic vegetables or high-quality frozen vegetables. Organic vegetables are typically higher in antioxidant and nutrient levels, all while containing fewer pesticides and toxins.
- Eat grass-fed, hormone-free, organic, pasture-raised, and wild-caught meats. Natural meats contain more nutrients, more anti-inflammatory fats (omega-3 fats), and less inflammatory fats (omega-6 fats). You don't want meat from a sick animal that is pumped with steroids and fed a toxic diet of grains.
- Eat healthy fats that promote ketones and the endocannabinoid system (MCTs, coconut oil, grass-fed butter, olive oil, and avocado oil).
- Eat natural foods that are low in carbohydrates, which will reduce oxidative stress and increase ketone levels to fight migraines.

See *The 3-Day Migraine Diet* for natural foods that will increase antioxidant levels with low-carb fruits, vegetables, sulfurous foods, B vitamins, vitamin C, vitamin E, and selenium.

That's it. Reduce processed foods, which will reduce the top food triggers. Use a migraine diary to track foods and triggers. Eat an abundance of natural foods, which will promote the endocannabinoid system and fight migraines.

Part V: Calm Body, Calm Mind

STRESS LESS WITH HEMP

This is my favorite subject in the book, probably because I'm a stress case when I don't continually practice the methods in this chapter. There, I said it. Hi, my name is Jeremy and I stress. Phew, I feel better now. Let's move on to why we need to battle stress to conquer migraines.

Oxidative stress is like a ravenous lion. Endocannabinoids are more akin to peaceful stoners. What would happen if you released a hungry lion into a room full of peaceful stoners?

Take note of the word "stress" in oxidative stress. Emotional stress transforms into oxidative stress.[280] So emotional stress releases this hungry lion, oxidative stress, into a room full of stoners, your endocannabinoids. That emotional lion kills your endocannabinoids and, thereby, kills your ability to fight migraines.

The result: psychological stress is the most commonly reported migraine trigger in research.[281]

Our Lions Are Not Real

A physical lion does not cause oxidative stress; it is the fear of a physical lion that causes oxidative stress. Unfortunately, our present-day lions take shape in the form of continuous stress from work, relationships, money problems, *mo*-money-*mo*-problems, or

163

that piece of crap who cut you off on the freeway because he didn't want to wait in the exit lane with the rest of us. He doesn't remember the event occurred, but you're still pissed off a week later.

When a lion attacks, a real lion, you survive or die. The stress comes and goes rapidly. When you have some unfinished work, you may go home with a low level of stress, go to sleep with a low level of stress, and wake up with that same stress level. Urban humans are stressing as if a lion is hunting them constantly, when in reality, those TPS reports that your boss wants you to finish have no real impact on your survival.

We need to break this stress pattern because indefinite stress leads to migraines.

Reefer Relaxes

Marijuana is a stress reliever. It relaxes the body, and after you smoke you don't care about those B.S. TPS reports that your boss wanted yesterday. Cannabinoids are a powerful way to stop the stress cycle that keeps you up at night thinking about something that's not a true life threat.

Unfortunately, marijuana may take this a step too far and make it mentally tricky for you to complete work. Here is where CBD from hemp picks up the slack. According to an extensive survey by HelloMD, a service that brings together doctors and cannabis patients, stress and stress-related conditions are a top reason why people use CBD.

Does CBD work? Oh, yeah. In my personal experience, hemp extract entirely removes stress and anxiety. My wife, Sondra, uses hemp extract to reduce the pressure from a fast-paced tech job that in the past would have triggered her migraines. The relaxing effects allow her to calm down, think more clearly, and get more done. CBD is like the older sibling of marijuana who is smarter, more prosperous, about an inch taller, and "why can't you be more like CBD," is what cannabinoid parents periodically ask of marijuana.

You need to try CBD to believe it before that oxidative stress multiplies.

A Pack of Lions

Stress is a lion that if left to roam your body will catcall other lions over. You don't want catcalling, as a once objectified firefighter, I can tell you that. Stress, anxiety, depression, and insomnia are a pack of lions and it doesn't matter which enters the body first, after a period of time the others will mosey on over.

It's not that a single lion is harmless, it might bite your head off, but a pack of lions encourage each other's violence. Stress, anxiety, depression, and insomnia are all strongly associated with each other and become dangerous when united.

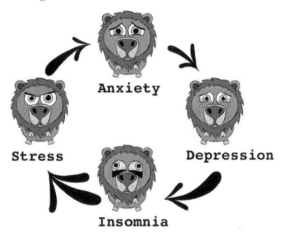

How do you think each of these conditions, which roll together, affect migraines?

Stress-related Conditions and Migraine:

Insomnia: A Korean study, published in 2016 in *The Journal of Headache and Pain*, of over 2000 people found that migraine sufferers were about five times more likely to suffer insomnia than non-headache sufferers.[282] Migraines make you exhausted without the ability to sleep. That's a form of torture. Migraines should be charged with war crimes.

Anxiety: Anxiety disorders, according to 2011 research published in *The Journal of Headache and Pain*, are also five times more likely in migraine patients than in healthy individuals.[283] You are probably thinking, "Duh, I can't work with a migraine and then I can't sleep. It's not paranoia if migraines are trying to kill me."

Depression: Depression increases the risk of migraine and, according to a 2015 study published in the journal *Neurology*, suicide attempts are 2.5 times more prevalent in migraine sufferers.[284] This is a sad statistic.

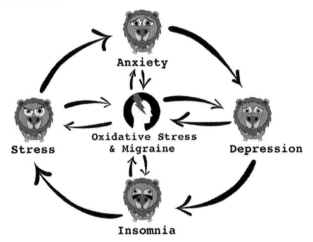

All of the above conditions, including their precursor of emotional stress, are associated with oxidative stress.[285] [286] [287] [288] But you knew I would say that, and you know that endocannabinoids will take one for the team and jump on that oxidative stress like it's a grenade.

We think of the stoner endocannabinoids, from my analogy earlier, as passive, but that's not true. Endocannabinoids seek out oxidative stress and say, "What a beautiful lion, I'll go and pet it."

The question is: Will using cannabinoids to spare your endocannabinoids be enough to treat the above conditions, as well as migraine?

Treating Stressful Migraines:

Insomnia

Although cannabis has been used for thousands of years to treat insomnia, research on CBD and restful sleep is in its infancy.

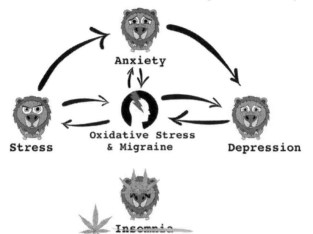

Many self-reported sufferers of insomnia, especially when it's from PTSD or chronic pain, have found that CBD has improved their quality of sleep. Anecdotal research confirms this notion and adds that CBD may improve REM sleep, which is deep sleep or quality sleep that is associated with dreaming.[289] [290]

I would caution that marijuana, with THC, will put you to sleep, but may reduce REM sleep.[291] (Note: The marijuana sleep research is conflicting and there are also studies of improved sleep for people with chronic pain.[292]) Any sleep expert will tell you that the quality of sleep is equally as important as the number of hours you sleep. For example, alcohol reduces REM sleep and that is one reason why you wake up after a night of drinking and feel like you never slept.[293] Some researchers are concerned that marijuana may increase the time you sleep, but unlike CBD, it may dilute your quality of sleep.

Hemp research suggests that CBD helps improve REM sleep and sleep in general, but user testimonials make it clear that there are some exceptions. Some CBD customers complain that they can't take CBD at night because it gives them more energy and keeps them awake. If you have a severe endocannabinoid deficiency, it makes sense that CBD will increase your energy by improving your endocannabinoid system. (Remember the mitochondria, the powerhouse that's regulated by cannabinoid receptors? Turn that energy switch back on and the factory will start up again.) If too much energy is your problem, try avoiding CBD at night.

I personally don't like using CBD at night because it makes me sleepy and I feel like pressing the snooze button the following morning. Sondra, you know who that is, likes to take CBD in the morning and at night, because it helps her mind stop racing so that she can fall asleep and stay asleep.

Sleep is more valuable than science understands. A new study found that chronic sleep deprivation builds up the amyloid plaque that is associated with brain lesions, Alzheimer's disease, and migraine.[294] We do know that improving your sleep reduces brain damage and migraines but we don't know exactly how sleep works or what sleep is capable of.[295] Trust that, while we may not understand why, nature knows what it's doing when it asks for a third of your day.

Sleep Pro Tip #1.

A recent study published in the *British Medical Journal (BMJ)* of nearly 200 migraine sufferers found that 3 mg of melatonin per night cut migraine frequency in half in a whopping 54 percent of patients.[296] Melatonin improves sleep and outperforms migraine medication, in this case, amitriptyline was outplayed. Do whatever it takes to get a good night's sleep, whether it's taking CBD or melatonin.

Sleep Pro Tip #2.

Blue light, especially from artificial lights and screens, throws off your sleep pattern and causes oxidative stress. There are apps, glasses, sunglasses, screen blockers, and light bulbs that block the migraine trigger called blue light, and help improve your sleep.[297] Feel good with a little hemp and look good with some shades that help hemp preserve endocannabinoids.

Those "migraine sunglasses," with their rose-colored lenses, work by blocking blue light, which can be accomplished with almost any yellow, orange, red, or rose-colored lenses. I'm really digging "BluBlocker" sunglasses because they take away all the eye strain from blue light and in my opinion, and according to the spectrum analyses from both sunglasses, outperform the blue blocking capabilities of $200 sunglasses that are marketed for migraine.

Get some blue blocking shades and avoid blue light from artificial sources, especially at night.

Anxiety and Public Speaking

A small study conducted in Brazil found that people who took CBD responded with reduced anxiety, discomfort, and brain fog during a public speaking exercise when compared to a group who took placebos.[298] Public speaking is a terrifying measurement of stress and anxiety for most people.

This study reminds me of beta-blockers, a heart medication used to treat migraine sufferers. Beta-blockers fight migraines by calming the body's response to stress and they are popular among public speakers. Many public speakers who panic at the podium take a beta-blocker beforehand to chill out.

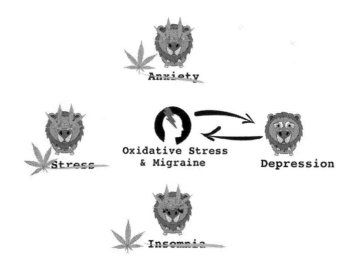

Blocking anxiety blocks stress and migraines. Maybe CBD and its ability to reduce stress like a beta-blocker will prevent migraine in the same way.

Depression and CBD

Research as far back as the 1970s shows that cannabis (both CBD and THC) increases serotonin levels, which is how most anti-anxiety and antidepressant drugs work.[299]

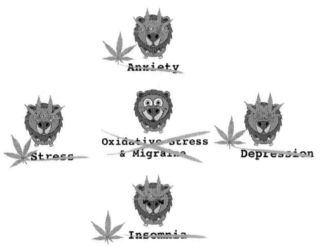

This initial research on cannabis's ability to increase serotonin and mellow out the body led to the development of a drug called triptans. Triptans, the first-migraine specific medications, interact with cannabinoid receptors and increase serotonin to stop migraines acutely.[300]

CBD combines the migraine prevention aspects of antidepressants with the acute ability to stop migraines in their tracks. What a chill pill.

Migraines are a Defensive Mechanism

Migraines are a defense mechanism against stress. Why? Why is it so damn important to reduce stress that the human body feels the need to cause a migraine? A migraine is a debilitating event that would increase your vulnerability to death in the wild.

Over 75 percent of all physician office visits are for stress-related ailments, about half of which are accompanied by some form of headache.[301] Stress is a major contributing factor to the six leading causes of death.[302] Stress-triggered migraines let us know, today, that long-term chronic stress can be fatal.

What should we do about it? Over 55 studies have found that biofeedback reduces migraine pain as much as powerful migraine medications such as ergotamine. [303] [304]

Biofeedback is a variety of relaxation exercises that are monitored by sensors that measure heart rate, blood pressure, brain waves, temperature, breathing, etc. However, according to Harvard researchers, you don't need all the costly monitoring equipment because simple relaxation exercises such as controlled breathing or meditation work just as well.[305]

Imagine if you combined relaxation exercises with the migraine fighting power of cannabinoids.

Relaxation Pro Tip #1. Breathe

Do controlled breathing for 10-20 minutes twice per day. A vape pen of CBD might be useful before this exercise. Also, doing a CBD-breathing combo when you feel a migraine coming on is a forceful way to stop a migraine acutely.

My favorite relaxation exercise is box breathing, which was developed to help Navy Seals survive BUD/S training.

It goes a little something like this:
1. Inhale for four seconds (don't inhale so much that it's uncomfortable)
2. Hold for four seconds (relax the body)
3. Exhale for four seconds
4. Hold lungs empty for four seconds (relax the body)
5. Repeat. Continue for at least 1 min, 10 to 20 minutes per day.

Or try Headspace: My wife's favorite breathing exercise is from Headspace, which is the most popular mobile app for meditation.

She likes that "it's really easy, the narrator has a soothing voice, and they provide different packs for say, anxiety, happiness, or productivity, and it is science-based as opposed to spiritually driven."

I'm asking her, right now, on a scale of one to ten, how much does it help? "Oh, ten, maybe 11," she replies, "They have rescue packs, so if I'm panicking, I'll listen to a 3-minute meditation, or they have sleep meditations that actually knock me out. I love it."

Breathe to help hemp relax the body and prevent migraines. It's a great natural addition to your migraine toolkit that is proven by science to reduce migraines.[306] [307]

Relaxation Pro Tip #2. Cold Training

In a new study published in the *Journal of Neurosciences in Rural Practice*, cold therapy reduced migraine pain and frequency by a lot, more than a lot, by a gargantuan amount.[308] When cold therapy was added to traditional medication, it dropped headache days from 10.65 to 2.0 days per month. When compared to the migraineurs who only took medications, people in the cold therapy group had less than one third as many migraine attacks.

The study attributed the migraine success to improved autonomic function.

Autonomic Function

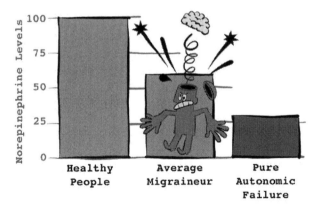

The average migraine sufferer has an autonomic function, measured by norepinephrine levels, that operates at only 60 percent of what a healthy person's autonomic nervous system should. Cold training improves autonomic function, the body's response to stress, and significantly reduces migraines.

Guess what else improves autonomic function? A study published by Oxford University researchers found that CBD enhanced autonomic function and reduced the body's stress response to cold, mental, and physical stress tests. [309] A typical test that measures your body's ability to respond to stress is placing your hand in ice water. The better your body can take on the cold, the better your autonomic function and ability to respond to all sorts of stress. You probably have the shivers just thinking about this because migraine sufferers have a weak autonomic system and therefore an inadequate response to cold and other stressors.

Cold training is known for relieving stress, anxiety, and depression, and for making you feel alive, which may be why it treats migraines too.

A well-studied method for improving autonomic function is the Wim Hof Method, by Wim Hof, aka the "Ice Man." You can also use a good cold pack or cold therapy machine. I use the Ossur Cold Rush Cold Therapy System with a Universal Pad, around the neck for 20 minutes per day. I can't go in depth here on all the science, since we're focused on cannabinoids, but you can learn more about cold therapy by reading my article on migrainekey.com titled, "10 Reasons Why the Wim Hof Method Freezes Migraines."

CBD improves autonomic function and the stress response to the cold. Do cold training to improve this autonomic fight against stress and migraines.

A Non-Stressful Conclusion

Stress is not one dimensional. Stress is interconnected to every system that represents your health. There are multiple ways that your body can become stressed, even if you don't feel it, and there are numerous ways to reduce stress, depending on where it comes from and how you enjoy relieving stress.

I walk for 30 minutes as soon as I wake up to reduce stress and

I also try to meditate, breathe, surf, and practice the Wim Hof Method as much as possible. You might find it's yoga or exercise that is perfect for your stress relief. We didn't even touch on how yoga and/or aerobic exercises are proven to relieve stress and migraines in multiple studies.[310] [311] Find whatever helps you relax and do it on a daily basis to save those endocannabinoids for migraine prevention.

In the meantime, CBD may help relieve stress or add to the migraine-prevention power of relaxation exercises, cold therapy, physical activity, and blocking blue light.

HEMP FOR YOUR BELLY

Nausea is the telltale sign of migraine, occurring in more than 90 percent of all migraineurs. When I was a firefighter, I thought a drug called Zofran was magic. A patient could be green to the face, but a quick-dissolve Zofran pill would have him or her smiling in relief within minutes.

Their smiles were not what I found magical, although it was nice, it was the lack of throw up on me. The research that allowed for the development of Zofran will give insight into how to treat the nausea of a migraine, as well as prevent migraines from occurring in the first place.

Block Serotonin, Block Nausea

Zofran is a leading nausea treatment for emergency medicine and made possible by cannabis research. Cannabis, with THC and CBD, has been used for centuries to control nausea and vomiting by blocking a particular serotonin receptor called 5-HT3.[312] Zofran also blocks this serotonin receptor. If you're thinking, *I thought we need more serotonin, why block it?* You are a smart cookie. Let's get into the deep cannabis research because it's mind-blowing.

Good Serotonin Vs. Bad Serotonin

Increased serotonin from the 5-HT3 receptor increases nausea, but the activation of a different serotonin receptor, 5-HT1, increases the serotonin that your brain uses as a happy chemical. 5-HT1 sends you happy serotonin and 5-HT3 sends you nauseating serotonin.

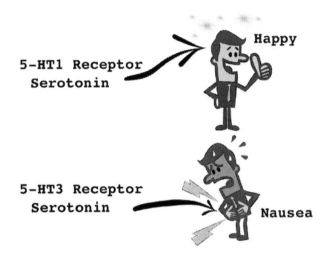

5-HT1 = happy. 5-HT3 = nauseating. Got it? Great. Both happy and nauseating serotonin will explain why CBD is your new best friend.

Cannabinoids Block Nauseating Serotonin and Increase Happy Serotonin

Cannabis has the rare ability to increase the serotonin for anti-anxiety relief and at the same time block the serotonin that triggers nausea. Drugs like triptans, ergotamine, and anti-anxiety medications are not so lucky and often increase nausea because they activate both serotonin receptors. Zofran is commonly prescribed with migraine medications to reduce the side effects of nausea. Oh, the irony. One drug was created to mimic cannabis's calming effect on the brain but came with side effects, so another drug was created to mimic cannabis's ability to calm the gut.

Prescription drugs that change serotonin levels are dumb, which includes prescription anxiety and IBS medications. They either block or increase serotonin, but your body uses serotonin in multiple ways. The brain conducts serotonin like a 60-piece orchestra playing an intricate melody, but medications act more like a single, hasty musician banging loudly on a cowbell. The body wants a beautiful symphony of serotonin, with orchestrated rises and falls in certain areas at certain times. But medications flood the entire body with serotonin. That's why the anxiety medication commercials mention suicidal ideation and diarrhea at the end, even though people take them to prevent depression.

Cannabinoids help the mind and the gut, a complex task that must come in part by stimulating the natural endocannabinoid system, which knows exactly how to conduct a symphony. The endocannabinoid system is responsible for controlling gut hormones, gut inflammation, gut permeability, and the gut microbiota.[313] It will all make sense in a moment but know that your endocannabinoid system is playing a symphony with billions of neurons in the gut and brain.

Nausea All Day

Hemp can acutely control the nausea of a migraine that is here, now. However, it's hemp's unique ability to improve long-term brain health and gut health that will prevent migraines from starting in the first place. Persistent nausea—like being seasick on a boat that doesn't stop rocking for days, even when you don't have a migraine—is found in 44 percent of migraine sufferers and it doubles the risk of developing chronic migraines (15 or more migraine days per month).[314] This nauseous connection comes from a direct link between the brain and the gut.

The Second Brain

Gut health is as crucial for migraine prevention as brain health. In fact, researchers have nicknamed the gut the "second brain" because it connects to the brain through an extensive network of neurons, hormones, and a highway of chemicals that influence our mood. The gut is thought to produce the majority of our serotonin, which keeps us happy and migraine free.[315]

IBS and Migraine

We know that migraines wreak havoc on the gut, but the relationship is a two-way street. Irritable bowel syndrome (IBS), which is vaguely described as any inflammation that results in "gut discomfort," occurs in more than half of migraine sufferers, but IBS also increases the risk of developing migraines.[316]

IBS and Endocannabinoid Deficiency

IBS may develop from an endocannabinoid deficiency, which IBS, fibromyalgia, and migraine patients share.[317] Anandamide, the bliss endocannabinoid, naturally activates happy serotonin, from the 5-HT1 receptor, and a deficiency of both endocannabinoids and serotonin is common in IBS sufferers. It seems strange that a lack of happy serotonin in the brain creates havoc in the gut, but I'll soon explain why we need both brains in tip-top shape for the body to feel happy.

CBD is a Breakthrough in Gut Relief

If a lack of endocannabinoids reduces good serotonin and wreaks havoc on the gut, what exactly does CBD do to the gut? CBD stimulates the 5-HT1 receptor to produce happy serotonin for the brain and is proven to reduce the gut inflammation associated with IBS in multiple studies.[318] [319] [320] [321]

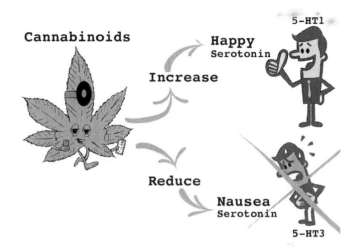

A new CBD chewing gum, produced by AXIM Biotech, was also successful in its first-stage trial for treating IBS.[322] Impressive.

It's easy to read through all the studies about CBD and become numb to how powerful it is. IBS is no joke. I have struggled with it and it's not fun. The brain and body do not feel ok when you have holes in the gut. That's literally what the inflammation from IBS does to the lining of the gut, the epithelial barrier. The gut barrier gets holes in it like you shot a miniature shotgun into all 25 feet of the intestines. This is called "gut permeability." This is the same "gut permeability" mentioned earlier, which the endocannabinoid system regulates.

IBS is not something that medication has been able to treat effectively. In fact, most medications are more likely to damage the gut, which will lead to low serotonin and a host of other problems. "It had been building up [IBS] for so many years, I just didn't want to live. I just thought, if I'm going to die, if I'm going to kill myself, I should take some drugs," said Kurt Cobain, the lead singer of Nirvana, in the interview that explained how IBS led to his addiction to prescription opiates and later heroin.

In fairness, after five years and multiple doctors, Cobain was prescribed a medication that helped, but he had already lost so much and died from a heroin-fueled suicide shortly after his tell-all interview. His experience is not unique: suicidal tendencies are anywhere from 3 to 11 times more likely in patients with chronic abdominal pain (the rate ranges depending on which study you reference).[323] Many IBS sufferers never find a medication that helps.

It makes sense. The gut makes the serotonin that makes you happy and people with a screwed-up gut are not so happy, which may be why migraineurs, 54 percent of whom also suffer IBS, are more likely to experience depression.[324] What if CBD could relieve IBS without major side effects? It would be, no, it will be, a game changer for many IBS and migraine sufferers.

The Brain and the Second Brain

New research on how the brain and gut communicate explains why each needs to be healthy for the other to be happy. Researchers refer to the connection between the brain and the gut as the *microbiota-gut-brain axis*. Abnormal brain function leads to inflammation in the gut, but it's bidirectional, an inflamed gut will also trigger inflammation in the brain.[325] This connection explains why stress is a top trigger of both IBS and migraines.

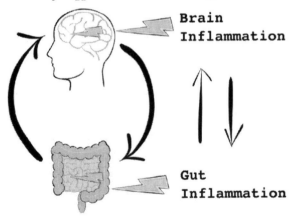

Let's say you are under chronic stress. Your brain sends an inflammatory message to your gut, your gut becomes inflamed and sends inflammation back to the brain, which gives you more stress, and the cycle continues until you overflow the headache threshold with inflammation.

Leaky Gut

Unfortunately, the inflammatory communication between the brain and gut is worse than it sounds, because inflammation is what increases those shotgun holes in the gut, you remember, gut permeability. Increased gut permeability, which you may have heard described as "leaky gut," is where migraine triggers come into play.

A Leaky Gut and Migraine Food Allergies

A leaky gut is linked to increased food allergies.[326] The theory is that an inflamed gut allows proteins to leak through the gut and directly into the bloodstream. Your body responds, "Ah, who let food in the blood?" and then creates antibodies to target the food proteins and kill them. The foods weren't a problem before, but now your body has antibodies to remember the food proteins, hunt, and destroy them. You then end up allergic to more foods, and those antibodies end up causing systemic inflammation throughout the gut and body.

A leaky gut could explain why one study found that migraine sufferers were allergic to eight times as many foods as the general population[327]. The list of migraine food triggers will grow as long as the gut is inflamed, making a migraine diet more confusing as time goes on.

The inflamed gut may block the absorption of vital nutrients for migraine prevention: water, minerals, vitamins, ketones, etc. Your brain may suffer the loss of serotonin because your gut is the creator of serotonin. Your body also won't be able to detoxify migraine triggers such as the biogenic amines found in aged meats, aged cheese, beer, wine, soy products, etc. A beat-up gut creates the perfect storm for developing migraine.

The Good News

The good news is that reducing inflammation can break the

inflammatory spiral that transpires between the gut and the brain. The best news is that the same research on the microbiota-gut-brain axis has found that a healthy central nervous system has the same bidirectional relationship.

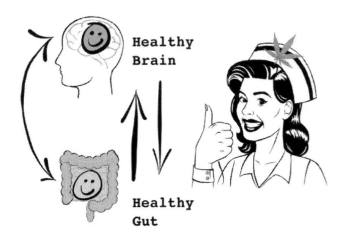

If you can increase the health of your brain, it will improve the health of your gut, and vice-versa. That's profound research, but you always knew it. You feed your gut healthy food, and your brain feels sharp. When you are emotionally ecstatic, your gut feels right, even if you ate Cheetos. It's a gut feeling that's bidirectional, and science can hardly explain it.

CBD is believed to control gut problems by controlling the neuro-immune system, which acts as part of the microbiota-gut-brain axis to interact with the nervous system and immune system. The neuro-immune system maintains the blood-brain barrier and controls inflammation.[328] Hemp also reduces mental stress, anxiety, and neuro-inflammation. This trifecta of improved gut and brain health suggests that hemp stops the inflammatory cycle between the gut and brain while initiating the healthy axis of a calm mind and gut.

We know that the endocannabinoid system controls gut health. Let's help the endocannabinoid system do its job with hemp. But why stop there? Why not do everything we can to control gut health, and thereby brain and migraine health, naturally?

Gut Pro Tip #1.

Peppermint aromatherapy was found in a 2012 study, published by Clayton State University, Georgia, to be more effective at treating nausea than Zofran, the powerful anti-nausea rival to CBD.[329] Peppermint oil blocks the 5-HT3 receptor, same as Zofran and CBD, and successfully treats intense nausea and vomiting after chemotherapy.[330]

Peppermint essential oils and peppermint oil capsules are no secret to migraine and IBS sufferers. Read my article "Peppermint and Menthol for Migraine Relief" on migrainekey.com to learn more about how to use menthol, the active ingredient in peppermint, for some serious migraine relief.

Gut Pro Tip #2.

Hemp and peppermint can help the gut, but if you are destroying your gut with migraine triggers, you may want to stop doing that. Easier said than done, I know, but a 2012 study published in the journal *Headache* may persuade you. The study found that migraine sufferers had a 44 percent drop in migraine attacks after patients eliminated personal food allergens from their diets, outperforming the majority of migraine drugs.[331]

These results are significant considering the diet did not remove common migraine triggers, sources of inflammation, or add in healthy fats and antioxidant foods. For a diet that does all of the above, *The 3-Day Migraine Diet* at migrainekey.com is designed for both migraine and gut health.

A Conclusion from the Gut

You didn't need this chapter to know how important the gut is. When you are happy, your gut is happy. When you are stressed, your gut is stressed. The research from this chapter only confirms what your gut already knew: a healthy gut will heal the brain and vice versa. Hemp helps relieve both stress in your brain and your gut. Get some.

Part VI: Hydration and Hemp

HISTAMINE, HYDRATION, & HEMP

Hydration is a painless and necessary way to help hemp fight migraines. Many people screw hydration up because they think water is all you need to hydrate: not so. Minerals are equally as essential for hydration and migraine prevention as water or hemp, which you'll soon see in the following eye-opening research.

Hydration is life. It's needed for neurotransmitters to fire correctly, for the filtration of toxins and migraine triggers, and for the absorption of all the nutrients that fight migraines. The whole point of using cannabinoids for migraine prevention is to reduce oxidative stress, inflammation, and glutamate. That can't happen without hydration. Dehydration causes all of those problems.[332]

The human body will last only three days without water and we, humans, wouldn't have made it this far without defense mechanisms in place. Migraines are one of those defense mechanisms, with dehydration being one of the oldest and most commonly reported migraine triggers.

Cannabinoids might ease the oxidative stress that dehydration brings, but if an animal were withering up in the desert, would you give it hemp or water or minerals? You want all three, but let's start with hydration. The following chapters show that water, minerals, and hemp are a powerful combination for the fight against dehydration and migraines.

What's Hydration?

We don't know what hydration is, or at least we don't know how to measure it. Science well understands dehydration, but hydration, not so much. There are varying levels of hydration and there are no biological markers that can accurately distinguish perfect hydration or even mediocre hydration.[333] Therefore, there are no studies that show how cellular hydration stunts migraines because there is no way to measure it. However, we know what dehydration does for migraines and it's not good.

Why Thirst Hurts

Histamine has an incredible relationship with endocannabinoids. However, to fully appreciate the endocannabinoid system, we need to understand how histamine both triggers and prevents migraines.

If you've ever run out of water on a hike, or in my case, run out of water while hiking on a wildland fire, you know that extreme thirst is an icky feeling. Icky, icky, icky. We have a biological urge to drink water and it kicks in way before dehydration settles in. This urge, thirst, is stimulated by the release of histamine.[334]

Histamine from dehydration is not meant to make you feel pleasant. The body produces histamine as part of an immune-system reaction to allergens. The same stimulus that makes you thirsty, histamine, is also what makes you feel like it was a bad idea to eat poisonous berries. For all your body knows, you are in the desert and may need to walk for several days to find water—but nowadays you're probably ten feet away from tap water. The body releases icky histamine to stimulate thoughts of survival, "I feel uncomfortable. Why? Do I need to look for water? Or maybe it was the berries I just ate."

Migraine sufferers know histamine as a biogenic amine and a top migraine trigger, found in many processed foods, such as aged cheese, cured meats, wine, and beer. The buildup of large amounts of histamine in the blood from thirst can trigger migraines in the same way as the buildup of histamine from processed foods or allergic reactions.

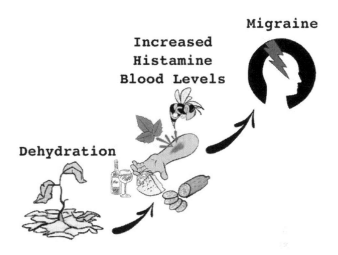

Here's where cannabinoids step in. Stimulating the cannabinoid receptors in the human body stops the histamine-induced itchiness, the icky feeling, that builds up in the blood from the exposure to allergens.[335] Brush up against some poison oak? Try using cannabinoid cream instead of that antihistamine or anti-itch cream.

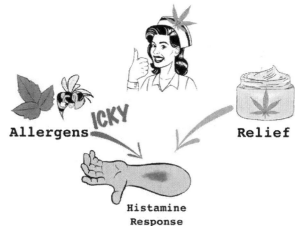

Oh, what cannabinoids do to histamine and migraines gets even wilder, but if you want to know why relieving histamine is vital, look no further than what happens to migraineurs during pregnancy.

Migraines Leave when Histamine Breaks Down

A study published in the journal *Headache* found that 79 percent of pregnant women stopped having migraines entirely.[336] If pregnancy were a migraine drug, it would be winning, at least temporarily. Women during pregnancy produce 500 times more diamine oxidase (DAO) than usual, which the body uses to break down histamine. On the flip side, women who have a genetic defect in DAO production, which reduces the ability to break down histamine, have a doubled risk of migraines.[337]

Note: DAO doesn't make histamine disappear. It is a process that helps the body metabolize histamine to get it out of the blood and into storage for a variety of uses—one of which we are about to discuss.

So, we know that histamine-rich foods trigger migraines, histamine from dehydration triggers migraines, the genetic inability to break down histamine triggers migraines, and migraines go away when pregnant women can metabolize histamine and get histamine out of the blood. We also know that the cannabinoid receptors sooth the buildup of histamine in the blood from those nasty, histamine-inducing migraine triggers.

Histamine is Bad, But Good Too

Most migraine research paints histamine out to be a migraine monster, but if histamine were utterly evil, an antihistamine like Benadryl would be the migraine cure for most. It's not.

Many migraine sufferers use Benadryl and it may work by controlling excessive histamine in the blood, reactions to histamine-rich foods such as wine (wine is not a food but you get the point), or by controlling the sinus problems that trigger migraines. However, antihistamines don't work for everyone, and completely blocking histamine can even trigger migraines.

This is another case where a drug blocks all functions of one compound, yet the body uses and needs that compound for multiple purposes.

Excessive histamine in the blood is associated with allergic reactions, seizures and migraines, but the brain also uses histamine to calm neurons, which may prevent seizures and migraines.[338] The histamine in the blood needs processing before it can be delivered into the brain and used for migraine prevention. Once inside the brain, the H3 histamine receptors release histamine, which blocks glutamate and calms the overactive nerves that trigger migraines. H3 receptor drugs that increase histamine in the brain are currently in testing for epilepsy, and if proven safe will most likely be used to treat migraines.

The problem with an antihistamine like Benadryl is that medications are simple-minded. Medications bang a single cowbell when the human body requires a symphony of chemicals at different times and in different places. If histamine in the blood triggers seizures and the histamine in the brain prevents seizures, what do you think will happen when we block all histamine?

According to the San Francisco Bay Area Poison Control Center, Benadryl increased the risk of seizures and accounted for about 7% of San Francisco's overdose-related seizures.[339] While Benadryl may block the buildup of histamine in the blood that triggers migraines, it can also block the histamine that the brain uses to calm the nerves and control epilepsy. If too much Benadryl triggers seizures, I am nearly certain it will also trigger migraines for at least some migraineurs. *Drugs are bad, M'kay.*

Got it? Histamine in the brain is good. Too much histamine in the blood is bad. That's why being prego is excellent for migraine prevention: it gets histamine out of the blood and available for use in the brain.

What if there were something that increases histamine in the brain and at the same time treats excessive histamine in the blood? Yeah, something other than getting knocked up. What if we didn't need to wait for scientists to create a drug that only knows how to play a cowbell, loudly, when there's a natural system that knows how to play a symphony?

Endocannabinoids and Histamine

You don't need to worry about CBD blocking the brain's histamine.

That's not how the cannabinoid receptors work. Researchers from the Queens Medical Center, Hawaii, found that cannabinoid receptors prevent mast cell degranulation, which is how the immune system releases inflammation and histamine.[340] The endocannabinoid system is not archaically blocking histamine like a man-made antihistamine drug would; it is controlling the immune system that releases histamine and inflammation.

There are different histamine receptors located in different places throughout the body. H1 histamine receptors are part of the immune system response, which opens up the blood vessels and causes inflammation, hives, and itchiness. This is the histamine in the blood that migraine sufferers want to avoid, which is associated with allergies, food allergies, asthma, and other migraine linked conditions.

CBD has relieved the histamine-induced symptoms of food allergies and asthma in animal studies.[341] [342] Cannabinoid creams also treat, both in research and consumer reviews, a variety of skin conditions in humans that result from a buildup of histamine from the H1 receptors.[343]

So, CBD helps treat histamine in the blood. That's all fine and dandy, but what about those H3 histamine receptors?

Histamine in Blood _Bad_

H1 Receptor

Itchy
Inflammation
Migraine Trigger

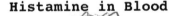

Histamine in Brain _Good_

H3 Receptor

Calms Nerves
Blocks Glutamate
Prevents Migraines

H3 receptors are the histamine receptors mentioned earlier that calm the nerves and may prevent seizures and migraines by blocking excessive glutamate. You can find H3 receptors primarily in the neurons of the brain and central nervous system, where migraine sufferers want histamine. Several studies have found that histamine from these H3 receptors can prevent migraines, and the development of H3 drugs for migraine prevention was proposed in a study published in the journal *Headache* in January of 2018.[344]

We can wait for new drugs or roll the calendar back to 2007 when researchers from the University of Washington made a prolific histamine and endocannabinoid discovery. The researchers found that stimulating the cannabinoid receptors increased the release of histamine in the brain, where H3 receptors play a significant role.[345]

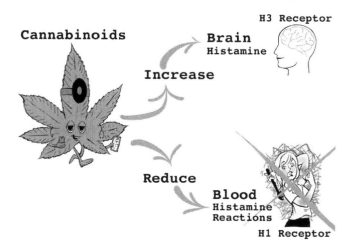

Endocannabinoids never cease to amaze: they treat excessive histamine in the blood (an inflammatory migraine trigger), and, at the same time, they increase histamine in the brain (where it is used to calm the nerves and prevent migraines). It's a double-histamine win for cannabinoids and their fight against migraines. Or you can get prego, your choice.

The H3 receptor is under research for the treatment of

Alzheimer's disease, Parkinson's disease, depression, brain lesions, MS, epilepsy, and migraine—all of which are linked by migraine.[346] However, it's difficult to develop a drug that can achieve what the endocannabinoid system does with ease, because the H3 receptor is complex.

The H3 receptor controls histamine with a feedback system. The more histamine released into the blood, the less histamine is released by the H3 receptor into the brain.[347] Got it? More histamine in the blood could cause less histamine in the brain. Wow.

Long story short: we don't want dehydration because it releases histamine in the blood and can trigger migraines. We also don't want dehydration because excess histamine in the blood may turn off the histamine switch, H3, that pumps histamine into the brain, where we need it to fight migraines. That clears it all up: histamine in the blood is bad and histamine in the brain is good. Dehydration is all bad for histamine and migraines.

The question is: what is the best way to hydrate to help hemp keep histamine out of the blood and in the brain where it can fight migraines? The next few pages will explain how water and minerals can fight histamine and a few other big migraine triggers. I don't know about you, but I am still titillated by the fact that the endocannabinoid system puts histamine in all the right places to prevent migraines.

MIGRAINE AND HYDRATION

While research shows that increased daily water intake results in a reduction of migraine hours per month, no migraine studies have added in the other part of hydration: minerals.[348] Minerals that dissolve in water or that are digested by the human body become electrically charged. Gatorade markets these minerals as "electrolytes." They are vital, but you don't need to drink a toxic bottle of sugar and food additives to get electrolytes.

Minerals from natural water and natural foods provide enough electrolytes to restore hydration even under the extreme circumstances of exercise-induced dehydration.[349] The problem is, most of us are not drinking mineral water that naturally flows down from mineral lakes or solely eating organic meats, fruits, and vegetables that have high mineral content. We drink purified water—because we don't want to drink bird pooh—that is void of minerals and we eat processed foods that require minerals to digest but don't replenish minerals, thus making us more dehydrated than eating nothing at all.

Migraine Minerals

You require five main minerals for hydration and migraine prevention. Without these minerals, the body won't be able to hydrate and you may end up with more histamine, oxidative stress, and glutamate than hemp can handle. Whether you get the minerals from natural foods or supplementation is up to you, but avoiding these minerals is not an option if you want to stay migraine-free. Say hello to **sodium, chloride, potassium, calcium, and magnesium**, or as I call them, migraine minerals.

SALT (SODIUM CHLORIDE)

Sodium is the most influential electrolyte for treating dehydration because it helps regulate the amount of water in and around your cells. Before you start putting salt on everything, you should check with your doctor if you have high blood pressure or are on medications that may conflict with sodium. The research to come will show that salt is more critical for migraine prevention than you would have ever thought possible.

Sodium Saves Lives

The need for salt to regulate hydration is why you don't want to drink gallons of filtered water in a short period, which has led to the death of athletes and even fraternity pledges during strange hazing rituals. Because you need more than water, paramedics use a mix of water and sodium chloride called *saline* to hydrate patients intravenously for nearly every patient in critical condition. Sodium chloride is salt. If doctors and paramedics use salt to save lives, maybe you can use salt for hydration and migraine prevention.

Salty Migraine Research

Research as far back as December of 1951 shows that migraine sufferers have an imbalance of sodium and may lose up to 50 percent more sodium than non-migraine sufferers.[350] Today, anti-seizure medications, which prevent migraines, work by regulating sodium channels to avoid overstimulation of neurons. Adequate salt intake does the same thing, naturally.[351] CBD also has this effect on the nerves but through different pathways.

Stanford researchers in 2016 tested the hypothesis that salt may reduce neuronal excitability and thus migraine. The study followed 8800 adults over the span of five years. They found that the odds of suffering migraine went down as salt consumption went up.[352] The regulation of histamine from proper hydration must also play a part in how salt consumption calmed the nerves and led to migraine prevention.

If CBD and salt both calm the nerves that trigger migraines, why not sprinkle some salt on your migraine fighting regimen? Salt will also help your hemp reduce another migraine trigger…

Salty Stress

Increased salt intake blunts our stress response, which may be why it's common for migraine sufferers to crave salt before the stressful event of a migraine.[353] Craving salt before a migraine is your body begging for you to relieve stress with salt. If you don't reduce the stress, yes, it may trigger a migraine, but it may also lead to a few other migraine risks.

Because your body uses sodium to block stress, people who are stressed out tend to have depleted sodium levels and the type of hormone deficiencies found in hypothyroidism patients.[354] Get this: sodium deficiency is more prevalent in hypothyroidism, and migraine sufferers are 3.5 times as likely to have hypothyroidism. Here's another crazy statistic that will bring us back to hemp: the majority of hypothyroidism patients also have depressed autonomic function, because hormones and sodium are needed to support the autonomic nervous system.[355]

It's eerie how all migraine research comes together. A deficiency of sodium will stress you out and cause autonomic dysfunction. Hemp relieves stress and improves autonomic function, which may be why it helps so many migraine sufferers. How about we use salt to avoid stress and autonomic dysfunction so we don't get to the point where we need hemp to save the day? Or sprinkle salt on our hemp, whatever works.

The Salt Myth

Salt was deemed unhealthy in the 1970's after the human equivalent of 500 grams of sodium per day induced high blood pressure in rats (the average American consumes 3.4 grams of sodium per day).[356] That bull freaking hooey research put Americans on a low-sodium diet, which stressed us the *bleep* out.

The salt myth, which suggests that a remarkably low intake of salt is healthy, has been disproven by multiple large-scale studies, that have found that restricting salt does not lower the risk of heart attack, stroke, or death in people with normal or high blood pressure.[357] Instead low salt intake was found to raise the risk of cardiovascular disease. Studies published in reputable journals that have followed hundreds of thousands of people from multiple countries have collectively put an end to the salt myth.[358 359 360]

There is no doubt in my mind that the salt myth contributed to the disaster of the fat myth, which peddled low-sodium and low-fat foods on us and pushed us toward many rapidly-growing-and-preventable diseases, which happen to share a migraine link. Hemp won't need to work as hard at reacting to cardiovascular disease and dehydration if those conditions don't exist in the first place.

Hydration Raises Blood Pressure and That's a Good Thing

If you added more water to the pipes in your house, the water pressure would go up. This is the same concept in the body. If you drink water, the pipes in your body fill up, and the pressure goes up. It's a healthy process. Your cells need sodium to hydrate, so the pressure goes up with a healthy supply of sodium and water because the entire body is hydrated.

When healthy adults drink too much water, we pee the excess out; same goes for too much salt. Studies show that even when healthy adults consume excessive amounts of sodium, the body uses only the sodium it needs and filters out the rest, just like it does with any other natural nutrient.[361]

When someone has a blood pressure that is dangerously high or is on a medication that may interact with salt, their doctor may tell them it's unsafe to stay hydrated with salt. One should listen to his or her doctor, but understand that salt is not the underlying problem with high blood pressure. Oxidative stress is the underlying problem with cardiovascular disease, and migraine too.

Oxidative Stress, Cardiovascular Disease, and Cannabinoids

We touched on this earlier and the following paragraph is a super quick recap so that you don't need to turn any pages, especially if your head hurts.

Here's the recap:
Oxidative stress is involved in the damage that occurs in the blood vessels, which tightens and restricts blood flow, and leads to cardiovascular disease.[362] CBD has been shown to reduce the size of blockages and increase the blood flow in animal models of stroke and heart attack. Plus, multiple experimental studies have found that CBD and the endocannabinoid system are beneficial in preventing cardiovascular disease by blocking oxidative stress.[363] [364] [365] Phew, hah, did you read that mouth-full of a paragraph without breathing too?

If cardiovascular disease is a concern that prohibits you from using salt, the endocannabinoid system can help.

Sodium and Endocannabinoids

Sodium shares a migraine link with endocannabinoids, but for that info, you'll need to understand how sodium and potassium work together to halt migraines. I'll also give specifics on how much salt you need per day, but after we discuss other migraine minerals because they all work together for hydration and migraine prevention.

POTASSIUM

Every cell or neuron has a door on it called the sodium-potassium pump, but I call it the migraine door. I initially had an entire chapter dedicated to this 7th-grade biology lesson, about sodium-potassium pumps, which I find more than fascinating, but my wife told me to get to the migraine point and sum it up. So, you can thank her for being able to skip the class, while still getting all the CliffsNotes on preventing migraines with superior hydration.

The migraine door, or the sodium-potassium pump, only opens at the appropriate time if you have both sodium and potassium available. Sodium and potassium work like keys, but with electric signals, kind of like a remote garage door opener.

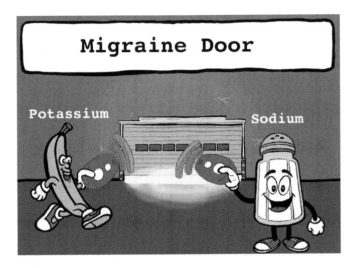

However, if you are missing one or the other of these keys, the electric signal will go haywire, and the entire cell will have an electrical meltdown.

Remember those Teslas? When too much glutamate gets sent too fast, the Teslas crash and cause an electrical explosion, which some people visualize during a migraine or seizure aura. The thing that picks up glutamate, those Teslas, before they crash is called a glutamate transporter.

Guess what door lets the glutamate transporter into the synaptic space to pick up the glutamate before it excites the cells to death and triggers a migraine? The migraine door!

The migraine door opens up to let out glutamate transporters so that they can clean up the glutamate, Teslas, before they crash and trigger a migraine. The migraine door is the sodium-potassium pump, which means you need both sodium and potassium to clean up glutamate and prevent migraines.[366] Class dismissed.

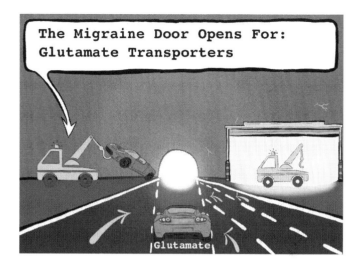

You want both sodium and potassium because they regulate glutamate, which you are also desperately trying to control with cannabinoids and ketones. Just out of curiosity, what do you think happens to people who have a genetic mutation that reduces the function of the sodium-potassium pumps? It's a migraine door, and people with a crappy migraine door are more likely to have migraine with aura and weakness to one or both sides of the body, which is called *familial hemiplegic migraine*.[367]

In contrast, migraine medications such as topiramate or amitriptyline block sodium channels to slow down neuron firing, which prevents excitotoxicity and migraines. It's better to calm the nerves naturally with minerals or hemp because hitting these complex nerves like a cowbell and blocking the sodium-potassium pumps can result in side effects such as slurred speech, psychomotor slowing, fatigue, and mental changes, to name a few. On the note of blood pressure, potassium is here to help. When people increase their potassium intake, sodium has *no* association with high blood pressure.[368] There's a sweet spot for optimum sodium intake, which we'll get to, but apparently, high sodium intake doesn't matter if you have potassium. A sodium study referenced earlier of over 100,000 people, published by the *New England Journal of Medicine*, also found that increased potassium reduced the risk of cardiovascular problems.[369]

The moral of the story is that potassium and sodium work together to hydrate the cell and both are needed to keep calm and keep migraine prevention on. Again, I'll give the "how to" and specific amounts of minerals needed daily after we hit all the migraine minerals because they all work together, as you will soon see with calcium.

CALCIUM

You are about to read some research about calcium that will make it look like an evil migraine trigger, and it can be. But there's a twist coming. As you read on, keep in mind that calcium is an essential electrolyte for hydration and therefore migraine prevention.

Calcium and Teslas

We know that when we send too much glutamate, or too many Teslas, too fast between the cells that they may crash. Endocannabinoids slow down those Teslas before they pile up on the freeway and trigger a migraine, which was the whole retrograde signaling phenomenon that was previously discussed. The problem with that analogy is that the synaptic space between cells is more like, well, actual space than a road. Teslas can't fly between planets or at least they couldn't when I first wrote this analogy.

Here's where calcium comes in. Calcium is like a rocket ship that launches glutamate, or Teslas, out of the cell and then releases glutamate into the synaptic space. I was wondering how we could visualize Teslas traveling between cells while editing this book, I kid you not, and then Elon Musk launched a Tesla into space on a rocket ship and released it with a trajectory toward Mars. Thank you, Elon.

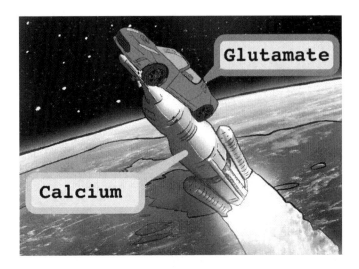

Calcium is that rocket ship that shoots glutamate, a Tesla, out of the cell (Earth) and releases it into the synaptic space (space-space) with a trajectory toward another cell (Mars). It's the same analogy where you have too many Teslas on the road and they pile up and trigger a migraine, except that we added calcium, or rockets, to the mix.

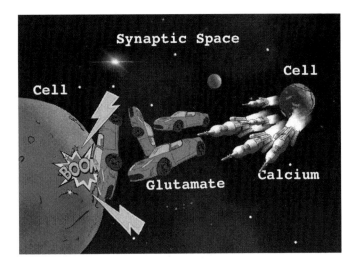

Just imagine that Elon launched hundreds of Teslas per second toward the same bullseye on Mars and they all crashed into Mars with a violent electrical explosion. (In real life, there was only one Tesla, which is currently off course floating through the galaxy.) Calcium and glutamate fly together, which means their levels are connected. Too much glutamate means too much calcium and too much calcium means too much glutamate, which means you will have too many Teslas launching toward the next cell, ready to explode and trigger a migraine.

If you recall, the cannabinoid receptors on the neurons are what slow down this process and prevent an electrical explosion. Here's an image to refresh your memory:

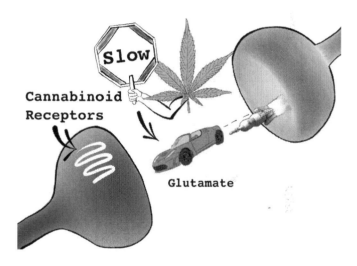

The electrical explosion from all those Teslas, glutamate, hitting the next cell is called depolarization or in layman's terms: the cell voltage goes out-of-whack.[370] Depolarization is the beginning of the migraine meltdown and will trigger everything that we are trying to prevent with CBD (e.g., overactive nerves, excess calcium, excess glutamate, oxidative stress, epilepsy, and migraines).

What do you think an out-of-whack cell voltage will do for migraines? *Hint: Hodor, Hodor, Hodor, hold the door.*

When Cell Voltage Goes Out-of-Whack

Remember that migraine door, the sodium-potassium pump? (I know, you just read about it, but some people are reading this with headaches and migraines and may have forgotten.) The migraine door is what opens up and releases glutamate transporters, which go and scoop up the glutamate before it builds up into a traffic jam, or space jam, and triggers a migraine. Well, the sodium-potassium pumps operate on electrical signaling and if you just caused an electrical explosion of calcium and glutamate (rockets and Teslas), that migraine door won't have the power to open.

The migraine door is for migraine prevention, but without electricity, it may swing the other way and let the migraine monsters out and into the body. Proper levels of sodium, potassium, and calcium create an electrical charge that will *hold the door* (aka *Hodor*) shut from letting out a migraine monster. (Yes, Hodor is an epic Game of Thrones reference.)

The migraine door is about more than migraines or hydration; it's the lifeline of a cell. Sodium-potassium pumps send electrical signals that allow your brain to communicate thoughts. An electric explosion from calcium will put a damper on communication, like shutting off the power to your brain's communication network. Silence at the cellular level causes cellular death, which is represented by oxidative stress.

Self-Amplified Loop

The goal of this book and hemp is to stop oxidative stress from spiraling into a migraine. It doesn't matter if the migraine trigger is stress from dehydration, emotional stress, gut stress, or stress from food triggers, they all amplify each other with oxidative stress.

A self-amplified loop is like when two people start arguing with each other and each person raises his or her voice above the other until they are both screaming. Have you ever seen communication get better when people start to raise their voices over each other? A self-amplified loop is a destruction that only leads to more destruction and there is no exception in the case of excessive calcium.

Oxidative stress causes an influx of calcium into the cell.[371] Migraine sufferers have high levels of oxidative stress and surprise, surprise, according to the data of 23,000 migraine sufferers collected by the International Headache Consortium, migraine sufferers are also more likely to have high levels of calcium.[372]

Here comes the loop: Too much calcium also triggers oxidative stress, which releases more calcium, which releases more oxidative stress, and so on until the body says, "Enough!" and unleashes a migraine.[373] As long as you calm one side, the other will follow. For example, if you gave a joint to two people yelling at each other, as long as one person smokes, the fighting will cease because one side or both sides will realize that yelling is not worth the effort and it's ineffective.

In the case of hemp, it relaxes both sides of the self-amplified loop by reducing oxidative stress on one side and calming the transmission of calcium on the other (we know this because glutamate levels correlate with calcium and hemp puts a chill pill on glutamate). Hemp is a two-for-one in migraine prevention.

Calcium is the Good Guy

A quick look at the calcium research makes it look toxic for migraine sufferers. Excessive levels of calcium correlate with oxidative stress, glutamate, and migraines. So, what if we had low levels of calcium? Would that fix the problem?

Clinical observations in epileptic patients prove that low levels of calcium are just as likely as high levels of calcium to cause nerves to become overexcited and trigger an electric meltdown in the brain.[374] The simple reason is that healthy levels of calcium regulate sodium channels and are part of the processes that maintain cell voltage.[375] Sodium, potassium, and calcium work together to support electric signals in the brain, which will keep that migraine door functioning at full swing.

Oxidative stress and damage to the brain cells were responsible for all of the calcium problems discussed prior. Excessive calcium only came after brain injuries, injuries which are found in the brains of patients with epilepsy, TBIs, Parkinson's disease, Alzheimer's disease, and now migraine.[376] Yes, all of these conditions are linked to migraine and can be treated with ketones and cannabinoids.

The research on brain injuries makes it clear that while calcium levels may go off the rails after injury, calcium plays a protective role in a healthy nervous system.[377] Calcium is the rocket that launches neurotransmitters out of the cells so that the nervous system can communicate throughout the brain and body. Without calcium, there's no communication among brain cells, and if you don't use it, you lose it.

The Calcium Take Away

Too much calcium from oxidative stress can be a problem for migraine sufferers, but this has little to do with the calcium you consume from natural foods. In fact, consuming too little calcium may increase mineral imbalances, dehydration, and voltage problems that end up triggering migraines. Consuming high levels of calcium from natural sources is less of a problem because the body will typically take what it needs and flush out the rest.

Cannabinoids, ketones, and healthy levels of calcium and other migraine minerals will help avoid migraines. As with the other minerals, we'll discuss daily recommendations of calcium with all the migraine minerals, because they do not function independently.

I saved the most renowned mineral in all of migraine research for last.

MAGNESIUM

I've said that all of the migraine minerals are critical, together, for migraine prevention, and they are. However, magnesium has achieved a level of success in migraine research that puts it in a league of its own. If you had to choose just one mineral to take with hemp, magnesium might be it.

It Started in the Nineties

A study published in 1996 in the journal *Cephalalgia* found that 81 German migraine sufferers reduced their migraine frequency by a staggering 42 percent after six weeks of magnesium supplementation.[378] One mineral had the success rate of the most potent migraine prevention drugs.

> *Fun fact: Cephalalgia is a strange name for a medical journal, but the medical definition of cephalalgia is "headache." You may have heard the term "cephalalgia" from "histamine cephalalgia," which is the old name for "cluster headaches."[379] Histamine is known for inducing headaches, especially cluster headaches, but research has also shown that migraine sufferers have extraordinarily high histamine blood levels, both during attacks and migraine-free periods.[380] Histamine plays a role in headache and migraine, so let's take minerals that reduce*

dehydration and histamine.

A study by the New York Headache Center said it best in 2012, "All migraine patients should be treated with magnesium." [381] "All" is the key word here. It's downright dangerous for researchers to use the word "all," especially for something as individualized as migraine treatment. However, the importance of magnesium supplementation for migraine prevention is now unanimously accepted by migraine healthcare professionals. And for a good reason.

Magnesium and Calcium

Magnesium regulates calcium.[382] Did your brain replay everything you just read on hydration and hemp? It's a lot to take in. I'm going to take you on a trip down memory lane. Just read the next paragraph fast and don't think about it too hard because your head will spin from the migraine prevention power of magnesium.

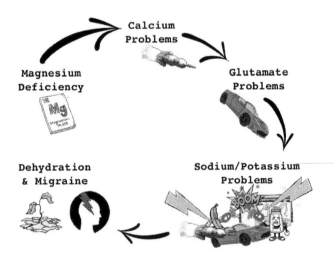

If you don't have magnesium to regulate calcium, calcium (rockets) will erratically shoot glutamate (Teslas) out of the cell and cause an electric explosion into the next cell. The sodium-potassium pumps (the migraine door) operate on electrical signals and don't function well with electric explosions. If the migraine door isn't working, sodium and potassium won't be able to enter and hydrate the cell. Plus, the glutamate transporters won't be able to go out and scoop up all of the glutamate (Teslas) that builds up between the cells. A buildup of glutamate causes oxidative stress and migraines. Hemp is used to relieve oxidative stress, but that's hard to do when magnesium, calcium, sodium, and potassium levels have all gone haywire and self-amplified levels of histamine, dehydration, and oxidative stress. My goodness, it all makes sense why magnesium is PubMed's top mineral for migraine prevention.

While all of the migraine minerals are connected, taking away magnesium is like removing the bottom three blocks of a Jenga tower. All of the blocks above will go down with them. Unless you're really good at Jenga, but even then, how many times can you poke the foundation of migraine prevention before it all falls down? Magnesium is, therefore, a requirement to keep the levels of all the other migraine minerals intact for hydration and migraine prevention.

Magnesium and Serotonin

Magnesium regulates serotonin. Migraine researchers speculate that this happiness chemical may be why magnesium can compete with the migraine prevention efforts of both antidepressants and triptans, which also increase serotonin.[383]

Serotonin helps control the excessive glutamate that triggers oxidative stress and migraines.[384] Plus, the happy serotonin chemical in your brain is the opposite of the feeling of emotional stress, which we know is the same as oxidative stress. Magnesium could push you toward happiness, which is more or less the same thing as controlling oxidative stress and migraines.

Salt Bath Anyone?

Ever heard of magnesium sulfate? It's Epsom salt, and migraine sufferers love to bathe in it. An Epsom salt bath is a natural muscle relaxer and stress reducer because of its ability to calm the nerves.

Pro tip: Take an Epsom salt bath and add sodium bicarbonate (baking soda) and lavender essential oil to relax the body further for migraine prevention or relief. Take a double dose of hemp prior, or get wild and take some cannabis oil with THC, and prepare your body for total relief. There are also many CBD bath bombs that include Epsom salt and lavender, which you may want to give a try.

Migraine sufferers naturally drift toward this type of relief, but the yearning for an Epsom salt bath must also stem from the body's need to replace magnesium, which up to 50 percent of migraineurs become deficient in during an attack.[385] However, this projection may be a gross underestimate, because routine blood tests can only measure about two percent of the body's magnesium since the vast majority is stored in the bones or within the cells.

Migraine researchers caution that all migraine sufferers may lack magnesium within the cells to prevent excitotoxicity, which a standard blood test can't measure. Excitotoxicity is the excitation of the nerves that trigger a migraine, which we are attempting to avoid by using hemp and migraine minerals. Don't be shy, take a dip in an Epsom salt bath and give your body the magnesium it needs.

Epsom Salt Migraine Success

Magnesium is the top migraine mineral according to research, thus far, but salt (sodium chloride) follows closely behind and may even surpass magnesium with more research. When we put both of these heavy hitters on the same team, balls fly.

If salt and magnesium are useful for migraine prevention, what would happen if you injected magnesium sulfate into migraine sufferers during migraine attacks? This experiment was carried out on 30 migraine sufferers in 2001 and published in the journal *Headache*.[386] Eighty-seven percent of the migraine sufferers were pain-free within two hours. If you're thinking that's a good success rate, it's not good; it's outstanding.

Only one-third of patients who use triptans are pain-free in two hours. Pain freedom is difficult to accomplish once a migraine has taken hold. Typical hospital emergency departments have low success rates for treating migraine and are blamed for prescribing the wrong medications, which end up doing more harm than good.[387] The most successful emergency protocol for treating chronic migraines, which includes magnesium sulfate, along with some other risky medications, is 97.5% successful at halting migraine pain.[388]

Magnesium sulfate is competing with the most popular migraine medications and improving the success rates of the strongest, and nastiest, drugs available in emergency situations. If you are eyeballing a needle and Epsom salt, just stop. Go back and read my legal disclaimer and talk to your doctor. We'll get to the natural measures of obtaining migraine minerals soon.

Epsom Salt and Cannabinoids

Magnesium sulfate has a secret weapon: it decreases CGRP in a similar way to the next-generation migraine medications. CGRP is the magnesium sulfate link to hemp, and it's a fascinating one.

We know that magnesium sulfate can reduce CGRP from research on Raynaud's phenomenon.[389] Raynaud's phenomenon is the pain sensation from unusually cold fingers and toes, which is four times more likely in migraine sufferers.[390] I've said it before, and I'll say it again, the consistency of migraine research pointing towards CBD is impressive.

If you recall, migraine sufferers have severely reduced autonomic function, which reduces the body's ability to respond to stress from the cold. The better your body can respond to cold, the stronger your autonomic function is for fighting migraines. That's why we Wim Hof it up, because cold training keeps migraines away and you won't need to say, "I hate the cold, my feet, my hands, so cold, all the time."

CBD improves autonomic function (our reaction to the cold), it reduces CGRP, and it reduces the oxidative stress that releases CGRP in the first place. [391] [392] Magnesium and salt are fighting the same migraine triggers as CBD.

Magnesium Summed Up

The research is crystal clear: magnesium is the foundation of migraine minerals. It supports all of the migraine minerals and attacks migraines with the same principles as hemp and the endocannabinoid system. The endocannabinoid system would not be able to function without this dominant migraine mineral.

I would go as far as to say that if Chuck Norris were a migraine mineral, he would be magnesium. I know, that's a daring statement to make considering how powerful sodium is for migraine prevention, but magnesium controls sodium. Let's not forget that back in '69, Chuck won the Fighter of the Year award from *Black Belt* magazine and his skills, and memes, have only grown stronger since. Magnesium is Chuck Norris.

However, if you google "hypomagnesemia" (low magnesium), you'll find that hypocalcemia (low calcium), hypokalemia (low potassium), and hyponatremia (low sodium) are all linked.[393] Migraine minerals directly affect each other's levels. Each migraine mineral plays a specific role in migraine prevention and none will succeed without the others. Chuck Norris might be the mightiest migraine mineral, but even he needs water and other minerals to use his 10th-degree-black-belt skills against migraines.

Let's get you those migraine minerals.

THREE STEPS TO HYDRATION

You're ready. You've read the research and know that hydration prevents migraines with the same principles as hemp. And you are about to combine them because you have the tenacity to kill migraines before they even look in your direction.

Or perhaps you just want to feel a little livelier, you know, proper hydration will also increase energy, nourish the skin, detoxify icky migraine triggers, sharpen the mind, heal the gut, and help you do whatever it is you like to do.

The following three steps will drastically improve hemp's ability to control migraines with the potency of all the migraine minerals combined.

Step 1. Eat Natural Foods

You could turn hydration into a complicated math problem and quantify every mineral in every food that you eat, but why go through the trouble? Your body does this elaborate calculation naturally.

It's straightforward: provide the body with an abundance of natural foods and it will take what it needs and flush out the rest. But we urban dwellers complicate this primal process with processed foods.

Rural communities that eat natural foods have a fraction of the migraine prevalence of their urban neighbors.[394] Why? Foods such as pasta, cereals, rice, and the hundreds of other packaged foods lack minerals and often add to dehydration because they require minerals to digest. Processed foods are like a black hole for migraine minerals. Rural peoples eat natural foods with water and mineral content, and we urban folks eat processed foods that take water and minerals away. Sure, this isn't the only urban factor contributing to our Western migraines, but it plays a massive role.

The simple solution: eat less processed foods and eat a variety of organic produce and meats—organic foods typically contain higher mineral levels.[395] The body does the rest; easy peasy.

Below are a few examples of how to get each migraine mineral, but don't stress: you'll find that most natural foods have some minerals and they all add up. Think like a caveman, or cavemadam, and eat whatever natural foods you find, civilly, of course. For more examples, see *The 3-Day Migraine Diet* at migrainekey.com.

Salt (Sodium Chloride)

Seaweed, Swiss chard, and cooked spinach contain high levels of sodium, but most vegetables contribute to your sodium intake.

Salt is a bit different from the rest of the migraine minerals in that we can add natural salt to our food, which is a good thing because many migraine sufferers are deficient in sodium. The human body has an incredible ability to crave salt when you are deficient and lose that preference for salt when you have a surplus of sodium.[396] So, listen to the body and salt to taste. (Specific quantities of each mineral will be covered in step three.)

I recommend natural salts, such as sea salt or pink Himalayan salt, because they taste great, contain other hydration minerals, and don't come with the unnatural anti-caking agents that table salt contains. However, I would say that I am a salt connoisseur; any quality salt will do the job.

Potassium

Spinach, avocado, acorn squash, and sweet potato are super high in potassium, but most natural foods contain moderate levels of potassium. The problem with most Americans is that we don't eat natural foods, not enough at least, so most of us get less than half of the daily recommended amount of potassium. Don't be average.

Potassium is the one migraine mineral that needs to come from natural foods. Potassium supplements are regulated by the FDA to contain less than 2 percent of the daily recommendation of potassium.[397] You couldn't get all the potassium you need from supplementation if you tried.

Don't be too upset with the FDA; there are health concerns from consuming an excess of pure potassium. Throw some pure potassium in water if you don't believe me. Ok, don't do that because it will explode. Watch a YouTube video of water and potassium instead, and you'll realize that natural foods with potassium are a tad safer.

Stop and think about this potassium conundrum for a second. Proper hydration and migraine prevention are impossible without potassium. The only way to get enough potassium is from natural foods, which very few Americans accomplish.

Calcium

Fish, greens, broccoli, sweet potato, carrots, and oranges are super rich in calcium, but as with other minerals, hundreds of natural foods contain calcium, and they all add up.

> *Pro tip: Your body needs vitamin D to absorb calcium. You can obtain low levels of vitamin D from certain foods but the sun provides the far majority (90%) of our vitamin D. Get out in the sun for a few minutes every day for the sake of your calcium levels.*

Magnesium

Natural vegetables such as spinach, chard, beet greens, seaweed, kale, cabbage, basil, summer squash, artichoke, spices and many other natural foods will provide most of the magnesium you need.

You want to get as much magnesium from natural foods as possible because large amounts of isolated magnesium can be hard on the gut for some migraine sufferers. Remember the most important scientific fact about magnesium: magnesium is the Chuck Norris of migraine minerals.

Get Minerals from Nature First

There are a bunch of caveats for the absorption of any given migraine mineral. For example, you need vitamin D to absorb calcium, but you also need healthy fats to absorb vitamin D. Don't forget potassium because potassium secretes stomach acid for the digestion of any mineral or nutrient.[398] But wait, if your source of potassium is from processed foods that spike glucose levels, you may end up with less potassium then you started with because glucose reduces potassium levels... oh, the caveats of hydration continue.[399]

I'll stop myself here. Tuna. Tuna is one solution that has all of the migraine minerals and healthy fats to digest them. You could also eat spinach and get a little sunshine to absorb all of the migraine minerals. There are natural options, plenty.

We could go on to find a thousand more caveats that will screw up hydration. It becomes easy to see how a single mineral won't do much for migraines. Yeah, magnesium proves me wrong with solid migraine research, but it's an anomaly, like Chuck Norris. And magnesium might help, but it is good for nothing if the other migraine minerals are truly deficient. We didn't even mention the caveats of all the other migraine minerals. However, something like tuna, or spinach, or a variety of other natural foods solve for all of these caveats. We don't need math if we follow nature's path—I'm such a poet.

The foundation of mineral absorption is natural foods. It's step one of hydration and we don't need to complicate it. Eat more natural foods and less processed foods.

Step 2. Drink Fluids

You've paid particular attention to how the endocannabinoid system fights migraines with migraine minerals. This combination is an extraordinary advantage that is idle without water, just as hydration is idle without minerals. So, let's get you that water.

The endocannabinoid system activates an antioxidant process that flushes out oxidative stress as if it were any type of waste in the body. Your body is about 60 percent water and without water, the body gets rid of waste, such as oxidative stress, about as well as your toilet functions without water, to paint a pretty picture.

Water is a necessity in transporting the nutrients that fight oxidative stress, as well as flushing out oxidative stress and its byproducts. After all, your toilet needs a system that brings water in and it requires a means to take... stuff away. But water is so much more than a transportation system, or a sanitary system.

Hydrogen, the "H$_2$" of "H$_2$O," is an oxidative stress scavenger.[400] Water will directly fight oxidative stress, as well as facilitate all of the transportation and sanitation needs performed by the endocannabinoid system. If you wondered how water could be such a great migraine preventive, antioxidant capacity is a considerable advantage, but it is just the tip of the iceberg.

Water helps control hunger, a colossal migraine trigger. Thirst is often mistaken for hunger. Are you hungry? Drink some mineral water and see if your body is mistaken. I don't call this a mistake— in fact, I can't think of any mistake that nature makes—because natural foods have minerals and water content. It only makes sense that the body makes us feel hungry to communicate the need for minerals and water... But let's not go down this rabbit hole.

We could go into how water helps migraine sufferers control hunger, the gut, energy balance, neuron transmission, and a long list of migraine triggers, but there's no time for that. It's time for action.

How many cups of water do we need per day? Search for this answer and you'll find many variations. Mayo Clinic suggests that women should drink 11 cups of fluid per day and men should down about 15 cups of liquid per day.[401] But what about the migraine sufferers?

A 2005 study of migraine sufferers found that increasing water intake by six cups per day, on top of whatever they'd usually drink, significantly reduced headache intensity and hours per week.[402] It's all arbitrary, isn't it? You and I know that there are no biomarkers for hydration, individual hydration needs vary, processed foods deplete water, and water is useless without migraine minerals. They, modern science, with current hydration testing methods, don't know for sure how much water an individual needs.

What is a certainty: most Americans walk around in a mild state of dehydration. Forget 15 or 11 cups of water per day or an extra six cups per day; the CDC estimates that the far majority of Americans don't get anywhere near the old recommendation of eight cups of water per day and 43 percent drink less than four cups of water per day.[403] We are water buffalo who migrated away from water.

So, again, how much water should a migraine sufferer drink? Enough to feel outstanding. Mayo Clinic's suggestion of 11 cups for women and 15 cups for men is a good number, so try it. Does it make you feel optimum? Or strive for an additional six cups of water per day on top of what you usually drink. Play around with the number of cups per day until you find what works for you on any given day. I try to drink water before every meal, when I wake up, before I go to sleep, and any time I need a little more pep in my step. That doesn't get me anywhere near 15 cups per day, but don't judge me, I'm trying.

Drink more water; the body will flush out the rest.

If you can afford the luxury of buying fancy-schmancy types of mineral waters, do it. Do it even if you used to make fun of people who drink San Pellegrino. The little bit of minerals in mineral water go a long way in helping the body get water into the blood and then into the cells, where the endocannabinoid system needs them for migraine prevention.

Drink Pro Tip #1.

San Pellegrino, Gerolsteiner, Vichy Catalan, or other mineral waters with high mineral content are incredible for hydration. I also crack some salt into sparkling water for taste. A pinch of baking soda can add to taste as well and help with nausea. You can also leave sparkling waters open for a few hours if the bubbles upset your stomach. Next time you take your hemp extract, drink some mineral water and write in your journal about how fantastic the combination made you feel.

Drink Pro Tip #2.

Stay away from sugary beverages. However, during a migraine or migraine recovery, you may want fluids that help you recover from low glucose and mineral levels. Sports drinks often lack certain minerals and contain far too much sugar. Pedialyte or coconut water are effective mixes of sugar and all the electrolytes that hydrate the body. They also feel incredible during a state of dehydration.

Step 3. Mineral Supplementation

As the name implies, a "supplement" is added to complete something. Supplements are not a substitution but an addition to natural foods and water. That said, electrolyte and mineral supplements can have incredible benefits for hydration and migraine prevention. An electrolyte supplement is something that is as pain-free as hemp and may be just the push the endocannabinoid system needs to control migraines.

What do I need and how much do I need? That's a migraine mineral question that I have thought about for years. There are a few things about hydration that we need to remember before we can succeed with migraine mineral supplements.

A few words about hydration:

1. There are no biomarkers for hydration and thus it is impossible to test for a perfect supplement. Supplement manufacturers guess which formula works best, which is why electrolyte supplements vary widely in mineral content.
2. The body needs all of the migraine minerals for absorption, so use a hydration supplement that is well rounded.
3. Healthy individuals will flush out excess minerals. Find a supplement with a healthy dose of all the migraine minerals and follow the manufacturer recommendations.
4. The need for supplementation will go down as you eat more natural foods and less processed foods.
5. Mineral needs can also change rapidly from exposure to

stress, such as physical stress (exercise), emotional stress, or migraines.

While mineral recommendations per day are guesstimations, research can help us avoid super low or high mineral levels. Guidelines become critical when supplementing minerals because isolated minerals can cause side effects.

Below are the daily recommendations of each migraine mineral. You know, the answer to your question: "What do I need and how much do I need?"

Salt (Sodium Chloride)

Multiple recent studies suggest that four to six grams of sodium per day are optimal for cardiovascular health and health in general.[404] [405] That recommendation may surprise you because some organizations recommend dangerously low salt intakes of less than 1500 mg of sodium per day. And we wonder why America tops the list of countries with the most unhealthy people: #Real1stWorldProblems.

Sodium is a powerful electrolyte for hydration and a little goes a long way in mineral supplements, but remember that the majority of your sodium intake will come from natural foods, mineral water, and salting to taste.

Keep in mind that salt is only 40% sodium and the rest is chloride. One teaspoon of salt is the equivalent of six grams of salt or about 2,400 mg of sodium, according to the CDC. You want at least four grams of sodium or 10.24 grams' worth of salt or 1.7 teaspoons of salt per day. Six grams of sodium is 15.36 grams' worth of salt or 2.56 teaspoons per day. Of course, natural foods have sodium and should reduce your need for salt supplementation per day.

Potassium

The daily recommendation of potassium is 7500 mg, but potassium supplements contain meager amounts. A potassium supplement might contain 90 mg of potassium, while half a cup of spinach has

420 mg of potassium.

You'll never get enough potassium from supplements. The far majority of potassium you get should come from natural foods, although the small amounts of potassium found in supplements are proven to help with hydration.

According to Harvard research, published in 2009, potassium is what allows sodium and water to leave the body and a lack of potassium triggers high blood pressure.[406] A lack of potassium may be partially responsible for the salt myth. In fact, high sodium levels have no association with high blood pressure when potassium levels are adequate.[407] As for migraines, a lack of potassium will cause an imbalance of all the other minerals needed for migraine prevention.

I know that you may be tempted to use a supplement for all the other migraine minerals and forget about natural sources of potassium. Electrolyte supplements help a ton, but for long-term migraine prevention, your body needs the vast quantities of potassium that only come from natural foods. So, try to nibble on some natural foods when you take your mineral supplements.

Calcium

The daily recommendation for calcium in the United States is about 1,000 mg, but it ranges among medical authorities. The World Health Organization's calcium recommendation is at least 500 mg and the United Kingdom's is 700 mg. What did you expect? We don't know how to measure perfect hydration, so medical authorities pull mineral recommendations out of the sky. It's all based on science, of course.

Any calcium supplement should contain more than sufficient amounts, with some going over the 1000 mg of calcium per day. Remember to take calcium with vitamin D3, which some supplements contain because that's how calcium is absorbed.

Magnesium

Magnesium is the migraine mineral recommended for all migraine sufferers. The men's recommended daily allowance for magnesium is 400 mg per day and for women it's around 320 milligrams per day. You can get more than this recommendation in the form of a supplement.

As a matter of fact, some migraine research has found that up to 600 mg per day will prevent migraines; however, a high percentage of patients suffered gastric irritation, most notably diarrhea.[408] You don't want poopy pants, because the gut is your second brain and you need your second brain free of distress for migraine prevention. Most migraine authorities recommend no more than 400 mg or 500 mg of magnesium per day to avoid gastric side effects.

Try a premium version of magnesium, such as magnesium glycinate, chelated magnesium, or other forms of highly absorbable magnesium. Premium magnesium supplements help avoid gastric problems. Although premium magnesium comes with a higher price tag, it's worth it for migraine sufferers.

> *Pro tip: "Natural Calm" is a favorite stress-relief drink, made of highly absorbable magnesium, which many migraine sufferers use to either abort or prevent migraines.*

What Supplement Do I Take?

We know that we need salt (sodium chloride), potassium, calcium (plus vitamin D for absorption), and magnesium. You may find that a daily vitamin of magnesium or calcium helps tremendously. However, sodium and potassium need constant replenishment and there are electrolyte supplements that can help with that too.

I like Saltstick Caps, which have high levels of sodium—many other popular electrolyte tablets have this important electrolyte too. Saltstick Caps are exceptional because they contain all of the migraine minerals, even vitamin D, and Saltstick Caps don't include any of the commonly used additives that trigger migraines.

Saltstick Caps are well known by athletes for preventing dehydration, and there are studies and research to back up this claim. Ask any Ironman competitor and they will tell you about a study that found that athletes who consumed twelve Saltstick caps during a Half Ironman competition finished the race twenty-six minutes faster than those who only used sports drinks.[409]

You might not be running marathons as a migraine sufferer, but your body is under stress that can add to sodium deficiency, which is more common in migraine sufferers. I believe that Saltstick Caps could be one of the most potent and easiest ways to help your hemp fight migraines. (I have no affiliation with Saltstick Caps.)

Some migraineurs will feel great from just one Saltstick Cap in the morning, some may want multiple electrolyte supplements per day, and others may need to combine Saltstick Caps with magnesium and calcium supplements. Again, the need for supplements rapidly changes based on things like how much stress you are under or how much natural food and mineral water you are already taking in.

Risks

Any supplement comes with risks. For example, some blood pressure medications can increase your potassium levels. Even common painkillers such as ibuprofen (Advil) or naproxen (Aleve) can elevate potassium levels. Taking a potassium supplement on top of medications can be dangerous.

For something as individualized as hydration, you should talk to your doctor and nutritionist about a winning game plan for natural and supplemental hydration. However, bring the migraine research mentioned in this book with you, because they might not know about the power of migraine minerals.

Hydration Summed Up

Hydration is not an option for migraine prevention; it's a requirement. Hydrate with natural foods and mineral water. Supplement when needed with salt (sodium chloride), potassium, calcium (plus vitamin D for absorption), and magnesium.

Try hydrating multiple times per day with electrolytes and see how you feel. Hydration could be the final push your hemp needs to get you out of the danger zone of the migraine threshold. It's also one of the most effortless ways to help hemp get you back to a happy and migraine-free life.

CONCLUSION

Congrats! You made it to the end and I hope that you learned so much along the way.

All of the migraine research that you just devoured, like a champ, boils down to a key concept: hemp promotes the endocannabinoid system, which fights off the universal migraine trigger called oxidative stress. Migraine sufferers have a low functioning endocannabinoid system and high levels of oxidative stress, which hemp helps fix.

Migraine prevention gets tricky because, as you read, the endocannabinoid system regulates homeostasis. The endocannabinoid system is responsible for your overall health and it's helped or hurt by the things that affect health, such as migraine triggers, nutrition, or physical and mental wellbeing.

While some people read this book and thought, "Oh, for F's sake, there are too many things that hurt the endocannabinoid system and trigger migraines," others saw an opportunity. The best of migraine research shows that the things that promote the endocannabinoid system are also the same things that fight migraines and we can combine them with hemp to get rid of migraines.

The research provides options and hope, and remember that hope is a good thing, maybe the best thing, in the battle against migraines. You might not need much more than a few drops of hemp extract, but it will come with the relief that you have an arsenal of migraine prevention options that work together to kill migraines.

But what were all of those things that promote the endocannabinoid system? This book covered a massive amount of research (look at the hundreds of PubMed studies in the citation section), which may be difficult to remember, especially if your head hurts. Don't worry; I've got your back. Don't let the teacher see, but I'm going to slip you the answers to all of the migraine quizzes.

To keep on track with all the inspirational research in this book, I've created a daily checklist and a guide to *Hemp for Migraine*. You can't put a price on migraine freedom, so I didn't. You can download it for free at www.migrainekey.com/hemp.

It's easy to set a book down and quickly forget about all of your intentions: Don't. Use the daily checklist and guide to give yourself the best possible chance of success.

I have one request for you. Oh, hold on, don't leave yet, it's a tiny request that would indubitably help me. Please write an honest book review on Amazon.com and/or Goodreads. I'd love to know, and other headache sufferers would too, what helped you, what didn't, or what kinds of info you think would help others in their endocannabinoid journey. You can also email me at Jeremy@migrainekey.com. Or, find me in the "Hemp for Migraine" Facebook group to see what's working for other migraine sufferers.

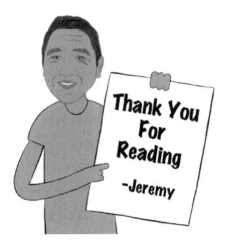

Thank you and I wish you the best!

End of Book.

Citations

[1] https://www.ncbi.nlm.nih.gov/pmc/articles/PMC3606966/
[2] http://migraineresearchfoundation.org/about-migraine/migraine-facts/
[3] https://www.ncbi.nlm.nih.gov/pubmed/26639834
[4] https://www.migrainekey.com/blog/how-much-does-the-average-doctor-know-about-migraines/
[5] https://migraine.com/infographic/migraine-is-more-than-a-headache-its-a-life-ache/
[6] https://www.google.com/patents/US6630507
[7] https://www.ncbi.nlm.nih.gov/pubmed/28775706
[8] https://www.ncbi.nlm.nih.gov/pubmed/25024347
[9] https://www.ncbi.nlm.nih.gov/pubmed/28861516
[10] https://www.forbes.com/sites/debraborchardt/2017/08/02/people-who-use-cannabis-cbd-products-stop-taking-traditional-medicines/#1a4a5bf52817
[11] http://n.neurology.org/content/82/10_Supplement/S41.003
[12] https://www.cdc.gov/drugoverdose/epidemic/index.html
[13] https://www.vox.com/policy-and-politics/2017/6/6/15743986/opioid-epidemic-overdose-deaths-2016
[14] https://www.npr.org/sections/thetwo-way/2018/01/30/581930051/drug-distributors-shipped-20-8-million-painkillers-to-west-virginia-town-of-3-00
[15] https://www.cdc.gov/vitalsigns/heroin/index.html
[16] https://www.ncbi.nlm.nih.gov/pubmed/28162799
[17] https://www.ncbi.nlm.nih.gov/pubmed/29019782
[18] https://www.nytimes.com/roomfordebate/2016/04/26/is-marijuana-a-gateway-drug/overdoses-fell-with-medical-marijuana-legalization
[19] https://www.usnews.com/news/articles/2016-09-08/fentanyl-maker-donates-big-to-campaign-opposing-pot-legalization
[20] http://news.gallup.com/poll/221018/record-high-support-legalizing-marijuana.aspx
[21] https://www.huffingtonpost.com/2014/01/14/marijuana-prohibition-racist_n_4590190.html

[22] https://www.ncbi.nlm.nih.gov/pubmed/9696453
[23] https://www.ncbi.nlm.nih.gov/pubmed/463911
[24] https://www.ncbi.nlm.nih.gov/pubmed/9696453
[25] http://bit.ly/2DWFopb (google book)
[26] https://coloradopolitics.com/despite-claims-data-show-legalized-marijuana-not-increased-crime-rates/
[27] http://caselaw.findlaw.com/us-9th-circuit/1253723.html
[28] http://www.ncsl.org/research/agriculture-and-rural-development/state-industrial-hemp-statutes.aspx
[29] https://www.congress.gov/bill/115th-congress/house-bill/244/text?format=txt
[30] https://www.dea.gov/druginfo/ds.shtml
[31] http://www.newsweek.com/medical-marijuana-cbd-not-addictive-toxic-who-says-748069
[32] http://www.ibtimes.com/marijuana-legalization-2016-deas-new-cannabis-laws-make-cbd-other-extracts-schedule-i-2460829
[33] https://www.fda.gov/downloads/aboutfda/centersoffices/officeofmedicalproductsandtobacco/cder/ucm498077.pdf
[34] https://www.forbes.com/sites/debraborchardt/2017/08/23/hemp-cannabis-product-sales-projected-to-hit-a-billion-dollars-in-3-years/#23c21383474c
[35] https://www.forbes.com/sites/tomangell/2017/09/18/california-officially-calls-on-feds-to-reclassify-marijuana/#600d3ec6427a
[36] https://www.ncbi.nlm.nih.gov/pubmed/28169144
[37] https://www.huffingtonpost.com/entry/jeff-sessions-state-marijuana-laws_us_59077dcde4b0bb2d087023df
[38] https://www.nbcnews.com/news/us-news/georgia-lawmaker-delivers-cannabis-oil-while-dodging-felony-charges-n752386
[39] https://www.ncbi.nlm.nih.gov/pubmed/26800377
[40] https://www.congress.gov/bill/115th-congress/house-bill/2273/
[41] https://www.ncbi.nlm.nih.gov/pubmed/26639834
[42] https://www.ncbi.nlm.nih.gov/pubmed/21518147
[43] https://www.hsph.harvard.edu/nutritionsource/antioxidants/
[44] https://www.ncbi.nlm.nih.gov/pmc/articles/PMC4818362/
[45] https://www.ncbi.nlm.nih.gov/pubmed/25024347
[46] https://www.ncbi.nlm.nih.gov/pmc/articles/PMC4969295/
[47] https://www.ncbi.nlm.nih.gov/pmc/articles/PMC2682269/
[48] https://www.ncbi.nlm.nih.gov/pmc/articles/PMC5241421/
[49] https://www.ncbi.nlm.nih.gov/pubmed/26129705
[50] https://www.migrainekey.com/blog/eliminate-migraines-three-days/
[51] https://www.ncbi.nlm.nih.gov/pubmed/12391374
[52] https://www.ncbi.nlm.nih.gov/pubmed/18644028/
[53] https://www.migrainekey.com/blog/eliminate-migraines-three-days/
[54] https://www.sciencedaily.com/releases/2017/09/170904093810.htm
[55] https://www.ncbi.nlm.nih.gov/pubmed/24814950
[56] https://www.migrainekey.com/blog/how-much-does-the-average-doctor-know-about-migraines/
[57]

https://www.projectcbd.org/sites/projectcbd/files/downloads/cbdpatientsurvey_september2015_carebydesign-6.pdf
[58] https://www.ncbi.nlm.nih.gov/pubmed/26749285
[59] https://www.ncbi.nlm.nih.gov/pubmed/19393844
[60] https://www.ncbi.nlm.nih.gov/pubmed/2146583
[61] https://www.ncbi.nlm.nih.gov/pubmed/29111112
[62] https://www.ean.org/amsterdam2017/fileadmin/user_upload/E-EAN_2017_-_Cannabinoids_in_migraine_-_FINAL.pdf
[63] https://www.ncbi.nlm.nih.gov/pmc/articles/PMC3997295/
[64] https://www.ncbi.nlm.nih.gov/pubmed/28861491
[65] https://www.marijuanatimes.org/the-endocannabinoid-system-a-history-of-endocannabinoids-and-cannabis/
[66] https://www.ncbi.nlm.nih.gov/pmc/articles/PMC4620874/
[67] https://www.ncbi.nlm.nih.gov/pmc/articles/PMC3997295/
[68] https://www.ncbi.nlm.nih.gov/pubmed/14526074/
[69] https://www.ncbi.nlm.nih.gov/pmc/articles/PMC2241751/
[70] https://www.ncbi.nlm.nih.gov/pubmed/28497982
[71] https://www.ncbi.nlm.nih.gov/pubmed/28783162
[72] https://www.ncbi.nlm.nih.gov/pmc/articles/PMC2903762/
[73] https://www.ncbi.nlm.nih.gov/pmc/articles/PMC5330095/
[74] https://www.ncbi.nlm.nih.gov/pubmed/18358734
[75] https://www.ncbi.nlm.nih.gov/pubmed/28861491
[76] https://www.ncbi.nlm.nih.gov/pubmed/28861491
[77] https://www.ncbi.nlm.nih.gov/pubmed/22832859
[78] https://www.ncbi.nlm.nih.gov/pubmed/20709233
[79] https://www.ncbi.nlm.nih.gov/pubmed/27086176
[80] https://www.ncbi.nlm.nih.gov/pmc/articles/PMC4852457/
[81] https://www.ncbi.nlm.nih.gov/pubmed/28169144
[82] https://www.ncbi.nlm.nih.gov/pubmed/29114823
[83] https://www.ncbi.nlm.nih.gov/pmc/articles/PMC4310259/
[84] https://www.ncbi.nlm.nih.gov/pubmed/19942623
[85] https://www.ncbi.nlm.nih.gov/pmc/articles/PMC3386505/
[86] https://www.ncbi.nlm.nih.gov/pmc/articles/PMC3165946/
[87] https://www.ncbi.nlm.nih.gov/pubmed/17959812
[88] https://www.ncbi.nlm.nih.gov/pmc/articles/PMC5655843/
[89] https://www.ncbi.nlm.nih.gov/pubmed/19896326/
[90] https://www.ncbi.nlm.nih.gov/pmc/articles/PMC3386505/
[91] https://www.ncbi.nlm.nih.gov/pmc/articles/PMC5265812/
[92] https://www.ncbi.nlm.nih.gov/pubmed/26577065
[93] https://www.ncbi.nlm.nih.gov/pubmed/21323909
[94] https://www.ncbi.nlm.nih.gov/pmc/articles/PMC2211386/
[95] https://www.ncbi.nlm.nih.gov/pubmed/25029033
[96] https://www.ncbi.nlm.nih.gov/pmc/articles/PMC3165946/
[97] https://www.ncbi.nlm.nih.gov/pmc/articles/PMC3001217/
[98] https://www.ncbi.nlm.nih.gov/pmc/articles/PMC4303752/
[99] https://www.ncbi.nlm.nih.gov/pmc/articles/PMC4993742/
[100] https://www.ncbi.nlm.nih.gov/pmc/articles/PMC3165946/

[101] https://www.ncbi.nlm.nih.gov/pubmed/28107775
[102] https://www.ncbi.nlm.nih.gov/pubmed/26748309
[103] https://www.ncbi.nlm.nih.gov/pmc/articles/PMC3165946/
[104] https://www.ncbi.nlm.nih.gov/pmc/articles/PMC3165946/
[105] https://www.ncbi.nlm.nih.gov/pmc/articles/PMC3165946/
[106] https://www.ncbi.nlm.nih.gov/pubmed/27487280
[107] https://www.ncbi.nlm.nih.gov/pmc/articles/PMC4887613/
[108] https://www.ncbi.nlm.nih.gov/pubmed/27418279
[109] https://www.ncbi.nlm.nih.gov/pmc/articles/PMC3165946/
[110] https://www.ncbi.nlm.nih.gov/pubmed/18072821
[111] https://www.ncbi.nlm.nih.gov/pmc/articles/PMC3824622/
[112] https://www.ncbi.nlm.nih.gov/pubmed/28720944
[113] https://www.ncbi.nlm.nih.gov/pubmed/18951339
[114] https://www.ncbi.nlm.nih.gov/pmc/articles/PMC2785529/
[115] https://www.ncbi.nlm.nih.gov/pubmed/16619365
[116] https://www.ncbi.nlm.nih.gov/pubmed/22127657
[117] https://www.ncbi.nlm.nih.gov/pubmed/22648222
[118] https://www.ncbi.nlm.nih.gov/pmc/articles/PMC5009397/
[119] https://www.ncbi.nlm.nih.gov/pubmed/26814264
[120] https://www.ncbi.nlm.nih.gov/pubmed/15257686
[121] https://www.ncbi.nlm.nih.gov/pubmed/19384265
[122] https://www.ncbi.nlm.nih.gov/pmc/articles/PMC4931881/
[123]
https://www.researchgate.net/publication/228604938_Stoners_eat_your_broccoli_Fol
ic_acid_enhances_the_effects_of_cannabinoids_at_behavioral_cellular_and_transcript
ional_levels
[124] https://www.ncbi.nlm.nih.gov/pubmed/23305292
[125] https://well.blogs.nytimes.com/2015/02/03/new-york-attorney-general-targets-
supplements-at-major-retailers/?_r=0
[126] https://www.ncbi.nlm.nih.gov/pubmed/25713056
[127] https://www.ncbi.nlm.nih.gov/pubmed/24739187
[128] https://www.ncbi.nlm.nih.gov/pmc/articles/PMC2503660/
[129] https://www.ncbi.nlm.nih.gov/pubmed/6250760
[130] https://www.ncbi.nlm.nih.gov/pubmed/6271822
[131] https://www.ncbi.nlm.nih.gov/pmc/articles/PMC3717338/
[132] https://www.thecannabist.co/2014/06/11/marijuana-questions-cannabist-qa-open-
container-law-enclosed-growing-outside-topicals-drug-testing/12961/
[133] https://www.ncbi.nlm.nih.gov/pubmed/15025853/
[134] https://www.ncbi.nlm.nih.gov/pubmed/16927957
[135] https://www.ncbi.nlm.nih.gov/pubmed/11993614
[136] https://www.ncbi.nlm.nih.gov/pubmed/27338837
[137] https://www.ncbi.nlm.nih.gov/pubmed/15464043
[138] https://www.ncbi.nlm.nih.gov/pubmed/17119542
[139] https://www.ncbi.nlm.nih.gov/pmc/articles/PMC4851925/
[140] https://www.ncbi.nlm.nih.gov/pubmed/28861491
[141] https://www.ncbi.nlm.nih.gov/pubmed/12477710
[142] https://www.ncbi.nlm.nih.gov/pmc/articles/PMC4251564/

143 https://www.ncbi.nlm.nih.gov/pubmed/20664830
144 https://www.ncbi.nlm.nih.gov/pmc/articles/PMC4550273/
145 https://www.ncbi.nlm.nih.gov/pubmed/20100298
146 https://www.ncbi.nlm.nih.gov/pubmed/15012666
147 https://www.ncbi.nlm.nih.gov/pubmed/29394166
148 https://www.ncbi.nlm.nih.gov/pmc/articles/PMC3612440/
149 https://www.ncbi.nlm.nih.gov/pubmed/22517298
150 https://www.sciencedirect.com/science/article/pii/S2210803316300033
151 https://www.ncbi.nlm.nih.gov/pubmed/25699012
152 https://www.ncbi.nlm.nih.gov/pubmed/20456191
153 https://www.ncbi.nlm.nih.gov/pmc/articles/PMC4310259/
154 https://www.ncbi.nlm.nih.gov/pubmed/19942623
155 https://www.ncbi.nlm.nih.gov/pmc/articles/PMC3763649/
156 https://www.ncbi.nlm.nih.gov/pubmed/20329590
157 https://www.ncbi.nlm.nih.gov/pubmed/27617709
158 https://www.ncbi.nlm.nih.gov/pmc/articles/PMC2824152/
159 https://www.ncbi.nlm.nih.gov/pubmed/27617709
160 https://www.cdc.gov/nchs/fastats/obesity-overweight.htm
161 https://www.cdc.gov/nchs/fastats/obesity-overweight.htm
162 https://www.ncbi.nlm.nih.gov/pmc/articles/PMC2665194/
163 https://www.ncbi.nlm.nih.gov/pubmed/1525798
164 https://www.ncbi.nlm.nih.gov/pubmed/12136063
165 https://www.ncbi.nlm.nih.gov/pubmed/25600719
166 https://www.ncbi.nlm.nih.gov/pmc/articles/PMC4307252/
167 https://www.ncbi.nlm.nih.gov/pubmed/26374449
168 https://www.ncbi.nlm.nih.gov/pmc/articles/PMC4000031/
169 https://www.ncbi.nlm.nih.gov/pmc/articles/PMC4887613/
170 https://www.ncbi.nlm.nih.gov/pubmed/29412125
171 https://www.ncbi.nlm.nih.gov/pubmed/22670794
172 https://www.ncbi.nlm.nih.gov/pubmed/18996873
173 https://www.ncbi.nlm.nih.gov/pubmed/23432189
174 https://www.ncbi.nlm.nih.gov/pubmed/27752226
175 https://www.cdc.gov/media/releases/2017/p0718-diabetes-report.html
176 https://www.cdc.gov/media/releases/2017/p0718-diabetes-report.html
177 https://www.ncbi.nlm.nih.gov/pubmed/21484568
178 https://www.ncbi.nlm.nih.gov/pubmed/26076890
179 https://www.ncbi.nlm.nih.gov/pubmed/27752226
180 https://www.ncbi.nlm.nih.gov/pubmed/26076890
181 https://www.ncbi.nlm.nih.gov/pubmed/29260593
182 https://www.ncbi.nlm.nih.gov/pmc/articles/PMC2699736/
183 https://www.ncbi.nlm.nih.gov/pmc/articles/PMC4941127/
184 https://www.ncbi.nlm.nih.gov/pmc/articles/PMC1325029/
185 https://peterattiamd.com/is-ketosis-dangerous/
186 https://www.ncbi.nlm.nih.gov/pmc/articles/PMC3951260/
187 https://www.ncbi.nlm.nih.gov/pmc/articles/PMC3620251/
188 https://www.ncbi.nlm.nih.gov/pubmed/25156013
189 https://www.ncbi.nlm.nih.gov/pubmed/15096395

[190] https://www.ncbi.nlm.nih.gov/pubmed/19393844
[191] https://www.ncbi.nlm.nih.gov/pubmed/2146583
[192] https://www.ncbi.nlm.nih.gov/pmc/articles/PMC4640499/
[193] https://www.ncbi.nlm.nih.gov/pubmed/22388959/
[194] https://www.ncbi.nlm.nih.gov/pmc/articles/PMC2680051/
[195] https://www.ncbi.nlm.nih.gov/pubmed/21375763
[196] https://www.ncbi.nlm.nih.gov/pmc/articles/PMC3721020/
[197] https://www.ncbi.nlm.nih.gov/pmc/articles/PMC4215472/
[198] https://www.ncbi.nlm.nih.gov/pmc/articles/PMC5078489/
[199] http://www.ofdt.fr/BDD/publications/docs/DCC2017.pdf
[200] https://www.ncbi.nlm.nih.gov/pubmed/19049574
[201] https://www.ncbi.nlm.nih.gov/pmc/articles/PMC1865572/
[202] https://www.ncbi.nlm.nih.gov/books/NBK98193/
[203] https://www.ncbi.nlm.nih.gov/pmc/articles/PMC3322307/
[204] https://www.ncbi.nlm.nih.gov/pmc/articles/PMC4294438/
[205] https://www.ncbi.nlm.nih.gov/pubmed/24854149
[206] https://www.ncbi.nlm.nih.gov/pubmed/24237632
[207] https://www.ncbi.nlm.nih.gov/pubmed/28538134
[208] https://www.ncbi.nlm.nih.gov/books/NBK98193/
[209] https://www.ncbi.nlm.nih.gov/pubmed/11416089
[210] http://www.alzheimersanddementia.com/article/S1552-5260(12)01499-9/fulltext
[211] https://www.alz.org/facts/
[212] https://www.ncbi.nlm.nih.gov/pmc/articles/PMC4809610/
[213] https://www.ncbi.nlm.nih.gov/pmc/articles/PMC4794845/
[214] https://www.ncbi.nlm.nih.gov/pmc/articles/PMC4988325/
[215] https://www.ncbi.nlm.nih.gov/pmc/articles/PMC3045545/
[216] https://www.ncbi.nlm.nih.gov/pubmed/21461357
[217] https://www.ncbi.nlm.nih.gov/pmc/articles/PMC3807029/
[218] https://www.ncbi.nlm.nih.gov/pmc/articles/PMC4950175/
[219] https://www.ncbi.nlm.nih.gov/pubmed/23493128
[220] https://www.ncbi.nlm.nih.gov/pubmed/16344345
[221] https://www.ncbi.nlm.nih.gov/pubmed/24612847
[222] https://www.ncbi.nlm.nih.gov/pmc/articles/PMC3241741/
[223] https://www.ncbi.nlm.nih.gov/pmc/articles/PMC3056006/
[224] https://www.ncbi.nlm.nih.gov/pubmed/23493128
[225] https://www.ncbi.nlm.nih.gov/pubmed/15670718
[226] https://www.ncbi.nlm.nih.gov/pmc/articles/PMC2844895/
[227] https://www.ncbi.nlm.nih.gov/pmc/articles/PMC3762736/
[228] https://www.ncbi.nlm.nih.gov/pubmed/27562529
[229] https://www.ncbi.nlm.nih.gov/pubmed/29093073
[230] https://www.ncbi.nlm.nih.gov/pmc/articles/PMC3716352/
[231] https://www.ncbi.nlm.nih.gov/pubmed/28053008
[232] https://www.ncbi.nlm.nih.gov/pmc/articles/PMC4598109/
[233] https://www.sciencedirect.com/science/article/pii/S2213453016301355
[234] https://www.ncbi.nlm.nih.gov/pubmed/15123336
[235] https://www.ncbi.nlm.nih.gov/pubmed/24413538
[236] https://www.ncbi.nlm.nih.gov/pmc/articles/PMC3620251/

237 https://www.ncbi.nlm.nih.gov/pmc/articles/PMC1865572/
238 https://www.ncbi.nlm.nih.gov/pubmed/18625458
239 https://www.ncbi.nlm.nih.gov/pmc/articles/PMC3116949/
240 https://www.ncbi.nlm.nih.gov/pubmed/29093073
241 https://www.ncbi.nlm.nih.gov/pmc/articles/PMC5685274/
242 https://www.ncbi.nlm.nih.gov/pubmed/21546126/
243 https://www.ncbi.nlm.nih.gov/pmc/articles/PMC5289988/
244 https://www.ncbi.nlm.nih.gov/pubmed/25024347
245 https://www.ncbi.nlm.nih.gov/pubmed/25125475
246 https://www.ncbi.nlm.nih.gov/pubmed/26853806
247 https://www.ncbi.nlm.nih.gov/pubmed/23436720
248 https://www.ncbi.nlm.nih.gov/pmc/articles/PMC5436333/
249 https://www.ncbi.nlm.nih.gov/pubmed/24380931
250 https://www.ncbi.nlm.nih.gov/pubmed/25237116
251 https://www.ncbi.nlm.nih.gov/pubmed/18801821/
252 https://www.ncbi.nlm.nih.gov/pubmed/27723182
253 https://www.ncbi.nlm.nih.gov/pubmed/15372606
254 https://www.ncbi.nlm.nih.gov/pubmed/15728303/
255 https://www.ncbi.nlm.nih.gov/pubmed/15985568/
256 https://www.ncbi.nlm.nih.gov/pmc/articles/PMC4211847/
257 https://www.ncbi.nlm.nih.gov/pmc/articles/PMC5214841/
258 http://www.neurologyadvisor.com/ahs-2015-coverage/migraine-prevalence-football-players/article/421162/
259 http://practicalneurology.com/2017/12/the-prevalence-of-migraine-and-other-neurological-conditions-among-retired-national-football-league-players-a-pilot-study/
260 https://www.ncbi.nlm.nih.gov/pubmed/24350853
261 https://www.ncbi.nlm.nih.gov/pubmed/25264643
262 https://www.ncbi.nlm.nih.gov/pmc/articles/PMC2652873/
263 https://www.ncbi.nlm.nih.gov/books/NBK209323/
264 http://www.cnn.com/2017/07/25/health/cte-nfl-players-brains-study/index.html
265 https://www.ncbi.nlm.nih.gov/pubmed/28687674
266 https://www.ncbi.nlm.nih.gov/pubmed/16829066
267 https://www.ncbi.nlm.nih.gov/pubmed/21443487
268 https://www.ncbi.nlm.nih.gov/pmc/articles/PMC4462058/
269 https://www.ncbi.nlm.nih.gov/pubmed/23886520
270 https://www.ncbi.nlm.nih.gov/pubmed/25732597
271 https://www.ncbi.nlm.nih.gov/pmc/articles/PMC5679535/
272 https://www.ncbi.nlm.nih.gov/pmc/articles/PMC5078120/
273 https://www.ncbi.nlm.nih.gov/pmc/articles/PMC4285050/
274 https://www.ncbi.nlm.nih.gov/pubmed/1908631/
275 https://www.ncbi.nlm.nih.gov/pmc/articles/PMC2846864/
276 https://www.ncbi.nlm.nih.gov/pubmed/16531187
277 https://www.ncbi.nlm.nih.gov/pmc/articles/PMC4247320/
278 https://www.ncbi.nlm.nih.gov/pubmed/18326600
279 https://www.medscape.com/viewarticle/886000
280 https://www.ncbi.nlm.nih.gov/pubmed/23490070
281 https://www.ncbi.nlm.nih.gov/pubmed/25160711

[282] https://www.ncbi.nlm.nih.gov/pmc/articles/PMC5052153/
[283] https://www.ncbi.nlm.nih.gov/pmc/articles/PMC3094648/
[284] https://www.ncbi.nlm.nih.gov/pubmed/26296516
[285] https://www.ncbi.nlm.nih.gov/pubmed/23490070
[286] https://www.ncbi.nlm.nih.gov/pubmed/22401887
[287] https://www.ncbi.nlm.nih.gov/pmc/articles/PMC3964744/
[288] https://www.ncbi.nlm.nih.gov/pmc/articles/PMC4596519/
[289] https://www.ncbi.nlm.nih.gov/pubmed/28349316
[290] https://www.ncbi.nlm.nih.gov/pmc/articles/PMC5101100/
[291] https://www.ncbi.nlm.nih.gov/pmc/articles/PMC4660250/
[292] https://www.ncbi.nlm.nih.gov/pubmed/24614667
[293] https://www.ncbi.nlm.nih.gov/pmc/articles/PMC4660250/
[294] https://www.ncbi.nlm.nih.gov/pubmed/25405649
[295] https://www.ncbi.nlm.nih.gov/pubmed/17883522
[296] https://www.ncbi.nlm.nih.gov/pubmed/27165014
[297] https://www.migrainekey.com/blog/why-blue-light-triggers-migraines/
[298] https://www.ncbi.nlm.nih.gov/pubmed/21307846
[299] https://www.ncbi.nlm.nih.gov/pubmed/5149894
[300] https://www.ncbi.nlm.nih.gov/pubmed/7672873
[301] http://www.apa.org/news/press/releases/2007/10/stress.aspx
[302] https://www.ncbi.nlm.nih.gov/pmc/articles/PMC3341916/
[303] https://www.ncbi.nlm.nih.gov/pubmed/17084028
[304] https://www.ncbi.nlm.nih.gov/pubmed/19935987
[305] https://www.ncbi.nlm.nih.gov/pubmed/19935987
[306] https://www.ncbi.nlm.nih.gov/pubmed/25041058
[307] https://www.ncbi.nlm.nih.gov/pmc/articles/PMC4600642/
[308] https://www.ncbi.nlm.nih.gov/pmc/articles/PMC4750306/
[309] https://www.ncbi.nlm.nih.gov/pmc/articles/PMC5470879/
[310] https://www.ncbi.nlm.nih.gov/pmc/articles/PMC4097897/
[311] https://www.migrainekey.com/blog/exercise-migraine-trigger-or-cure/
[312] https://www.ncbi.nlm.nih.gov/pubmed/21477640
[313] https://www.ncbi.nlm.nih.gov/pmc/articles/PMC4940133/
[314] https://www.ncbi.nlm.nih.gov/pubmed/25250833
[315] https://www.scientificamerican.com/article/gut-feelings-the-second-brain-in-our-gastrointestinal-systems-excerpt/
[316] https://www.ncbi.nlm.nih.gov/pubmed/24838228
[317] https://www.ncbi.nlm.nih.gov/pubmed/18404144
[318] https://www.ncbi.nlm.nih.gov/pubmed/22163000
[319] https://www.ncbi.nlm.nih.gov/pubmed/22815234
[320] https://www.ncbi.nlm.nih.gov/pubmed/21726418
[321] https://www.ncbi.nlm.nih.gov/pubmed/20117132
[322] https://globenewswire.com/news-release/2017/11/21/1198101/0/en/Axim-Biotechnologies-Announces-Phase-IIa-Trial-Results-Validating-its-Proprietary-Cannabinoid-Delivery-Method-for-Treatment-of-Irritable-Bowel-Syndrome-IBS.html
[323] https://www.ncbi.nlm.nih.gov/pubmed/17593064
[324] https://www.sciencedaily.com/releases/2016/02/160223171421.htm
[325] https://www.ncbi.nlm.nih.gov/pmc/articles/PMC4240046/

[326] https://www.ncbi.nlm.nih.gov/pubmed/21070397/
[327] https://www.ncbi.nlm.nih.gov/pubmed/18693538
[328] https://www.ncbi.nlm.nih.gov/pubmed/22163000
[329] https://www.ncbi.nlm.nih.gov/pubmed/22034523
[330] https://www.ncbi.nlm.nih.gov/pmc/articles/PMC3562057/
[331] https://www.ncbi.nlm.nih.gov/pubmed/23216231
[332] https://www.migrainekey.com/migraine-trigger/dehydration/
[333] https://www.ncbi.nlm.nih.gov/pmc/articles/PMC2908954/
[334] https://www.ncbi.nlm.nih.gov/pubmed/11164999
[335] https://www.ncbi.nlm.nih.gov/pubmed/12835895
[336] https://www.ncbi.nlm.nih.gov/pubmed/16618254
[337] https://www.ncbi.nlm.nih.gov/pubmed/25612138
[338] https://www.ncbi.nlm.nih.gov/pmc/articles/PMC3514756/
[339] https://www.ncbi.nlm.nih.gov/pubmed/22742831
[340] https://www.ncbi.nlm.nih.gov/pmc/articles/PMC1138953/
[341] https://www.ncbi.nlm.nih.gov/pubmed/23428645
[342] https://www.ncbi.nlm.nih.gov/pmc/articles/PMC4458548/
[343] https://www.ncbi.nlm.nih.gov/pubmed/28416341
[344] https://www.ncbi.nlm.nih.gov/pubmed/28862769
[345] https://www.ncbi.nlm.nih.gov/pmc/articles/PMC1769340/
[346] https://www.ncbi.nlm.nih.gov/pubmed/27303254
[347] https://www.ncbi.nlm.nih.gov/pubmed/2172771
[348] https://www.ncbi.nlm.nih.gov/pubmed/16128874
[349] https://www.ncbi.nlm.nih.gov/pubmed/8781863
[350] https://www.ncbi.nlm.nih.gov/pmc/articles/PMC2070698/
[351] https://www.ncbi.nlm.nih.gov/pubmed/9435180
[352] https://www.ncbi.nlm.nih.gov/pubmed/27016121
[353] https://www.ncbi.nlm.nih.gov/pubmed/21471383
[354] https://www.ncbi.nlm.nih.gov/pmc/articles/PMC3183532/
[355] https://www.migrainekey.com/migraine-prevention/salt-hydration-migraine-prevention/
[356] https://www.scientificamerican.com/article/its-time-to-end-the-war-on-salt/
[357] https://www.migrainekey.com/migraine-prevention/salt-hydration-migraine-prevention/
[358] https://www.ncbi.nlm.nih.gov/pubmed/22110105
[359] https://www.ncbi.nlm.nih.gov/pubmed/25119607
[360] https://www.ncbi.nlm.nih.gov/pubmed/27216139
[361] https://www.ncbi.nlm.nih.gov/pubmed/733808
[362] https://www.ncbi.nlm.nih.gov/pubmed/20361706
[363] https://www.ncbi.nlm.nih.gov/pmc/articles/PMC4941127/
[364] https://www.ncbi.nlm.nih.gov/pubmed/22503477
[365] https://www.ncbi.nlm.nih.gov/pubmed/22670794
[366] https://www.ncbi.nlm.nih.gov/pubmed/19553454
[367] https://www.ncbi.nlm.nih.gov/pubmed/21731499
[368] https://www.ncbi.nlm.nih.gov/pubmed/24524886
[369] https://www.ncbi.nlm.nih.gov/pubmed/25119607
[370] https://www.ncbi.nlm.nih.gov/pubmed/17483292

[371] https://www.ncbi.nlm.nih.gov/pubmed/11841831
[372] https://www.ncbi.nlm.nih.gov/pubmed/20649555
[373] https://www.ncbi.nlm.nih.gov/pubmed/20649555
[374] https://www.ncbi.nlm.nih.gov/pmc/articles/PMC4374060/
[375] https://www.ncbi.nlm.nih.gov/pubmed/10097179
[376] https://www.ncbi.nlm.nih.gov/pmc/articles/PMC3324969/
[377] https://www.ncbi.nlm.nih.gov/pmc/articles/PMC3324969/
[378] https://www.ncbi.nlm.nih.gov/pubmed/8792038
[379] https://www.ncbi.nlm.nih.gov/pmc/articles/PMC3476069/
[380] https://www.ncbi.nlm.nih.gov/pubmed/12641658
[381] https://www.ncbi.nlm.nih.gov/pubmed/22426836
[382] https://www.ncbi.nlm.nih.gov/pubmed/19271946
[383] https://www.ncbi.nlm.nih.gov/pubmed/19271946
[384] https://www.ncbi.nlm.nih.gov/pmc/articles/PMC3968911/
[385] https://www.ncbi.nlm.nih.gov/pubmed/9523054
[386] https://www.ncbi.nlm.nih.gov/pubmed/11251702
[387] https://www.ncbi.nlm.nih.gov/pmc/articles/PMC3737484/
[388] https://www.ncbi.nlm.nih.gov/pubmed/16499830
[389] https://www.ncbi.nlm.nih.gov/pubmed/7820978
[390] https://www.ncbi.nlm.nih.gov/pubmed/25776043
[391] https://www.ncbi.nlm.nih.gov/pmc/articles/PMC5470879/
[392] https://www.ncbi.nlm.nih.gov/pmc/articles/PMC4851925/
[393] https://www.ncbi.nlm.nih.gov/pubmed/6476998
[394] https://www.ncbi.nlm.nih.gov/pubmed/24814950
[395] https://www.ncbi.nlm.nih.gov/pubmed/11327522
[396] https://www.ncbi.nlm.nih.gov/pmc/articles/PMC2908954/
[397] https://www.health.harvard.edu/staying-healthy/should-i-take-a-potassium-supplement
[398] https://www.ncbi.nlm.nih.gov/pmc/articles/PMC3197792/
[399] https://www.ncbi.nlm.nih.gov/pmc/articles/PMC4622792/
[400] https://www.ncbi.nlm.nih.gov/pmc/articles/PMC3563451/
[401] https://www.mayoclinic.org/healthy-lifestyle/nutrition-and-healthy-eating/in-depth/water/art-20044256
[402] https://www.ncbi.nlm.nih.gov/pubmed/16128874
[403] https://www.cdc.gov/pcd/issues/2013/12_0248.htm
[404] https://www.ncbi.nlm.nih.gov/pubmed/25119607
[405] https://www.ncbi.nlm.nih.gov/pubmed/27216139
[406] https://www.health.harvard.edu/newsletter_article/Potassium_and_sodium_out_of_balance
[407] https://www.ncbi.nlm.nih.gov/pubmed/24524886
[408] https://www.ncbi.nlm.nih.gov/pubmed/8792038
[409] https://www.ncbi.nlm.nih.gov/pubmed/25683094

Made in the USA
Monee, IL
24 February 2021

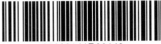

61230141R00140